The family on our cover is 'lost' because they're going to the hospital to see their Mom, who's not only very ill – she's in Intensive Care. They're all frightened silly. Mom is the bulwark of their family, and she became ill so suddenly! And yes, she is young enough to have small children.

Should you ever find yourself in this position where Mom – or Dad, Gramma or Gramps – or even one of the kids ends up in Intensive Care, this book will help you care for yourself first, and then your loved one.

It's the book you should have – and keep – for that scary time . . . just in case.

An Intensive Care Guide For the Family

A resource for families of patients
in the intensive care unit

Javier Provencio, MD
and
Kelly Ferjutz

2014

An Intensive Care Guide For the Family

© 2014 J. Javier Provencio, MD, and
  Kelly Ferjutz
Cover art by Alex, Olivia and Ben Provencio
  © 2014

ISBN-13: 978-1499662771
ISBN-10: 1499662777

This book is also published as an e-book through Kindle. The ASIN number is: B00KIXZHS4

All rights reserved. This material may not be reproduced in whole or part by any means, electronically or in print, without written permission from the authors.

Acknowledgements

I would like to thank Paul Ford and Heather Mekesa for reviewing parts of the manuscript. I would also like to thank my colleagues in the ICU (physicians, nurses, and all the other people who make the ICU work). I would like to thank the patients I have cared for who have allowed me to be part of their lives during the scariest times they experience. I would like to thank Kelly Ferjutz for being a great team-mate and offering her personal experiences with her own mother and daughter; and for pushing me to complete and publish this book.

I also owe a debt of gratitude to Kevin Mooney for helping to navigate the legal issues around the book that were part of this journey.

Finally, I would like to thank and dedicate this book to my wife Samantha. It is because of her love that I can work long days, experience heartaches with patients and their families, and come home to my safe place with my family.
Javier Provencio

Working with a physician who takes the time to explain things so that anyone can understand is a rare pleasure. I am grateful for the patience and knowledge of Javier Provencio, which he so willingly shared with me during this process. If we have answered one question for one family – it will have been worth it!
Kelly Ferjutz

As a convention, Kelly Ferjutz and Javier Provencio will refer to ourselves in the first person (I as opposed to we). It makes the book read more easily and makes it less confusing trying to figure out who is referring to what. Suffice it to say, all of the information in this book comes from a close collaboration between us. Even we can't always figure out who is saying what. *We* will be reserved for times when we're talking about the ICU community as a whole.

Resources mentioned in this book:

www.myicucare.org Critical care general for families
http://www.aacn.org/wd/publishing/docs/pressroom/icutip.pdf Tips from/about nursing
www.uslivingwillregistry.com Living wills
http://www.capc.org/ipal/ipal-icu/patient-family-resources Palliative care options
http://www.shareyourlife.org Organ Donation options.

Please visit our web-site for comments and/or questions: www.intensivecareguidebook.com

Table of Contents

Introduction
A Note on Progress in the ICU
But first -- meet the Browns
Glossary
Types of ICUs
Things you find in ICU rooms
Types of tests done in the ICU
Therapies found in ICUs
Two terms to understand

Chapter 1   The First 12 Hours
A very bad day for the Browns
Making sense of the first 12 hours
Wanting to know prognosis
Setting up a home base and establishing your 'team'
Limiting Outside Conjecture
Worksheet 1

Chapter 2   Meet the ICU Team
Alex Brown meets the health care team
Who is on your healthcare team- the history
The care team
   Physicians
The patient's primary doctor
   The Intensivist – whose specialty IS the ICU
   The consulting specialists
   (There may also be Residents and Fellows)
   Nurses
   Registered nurses (RN)
   Licensed practical nurses (LPN)
   Clinical technicians (CT)
   Non-physician care practitioners

Physician Assistant (PA)
Nurse Practitioner (NP)
Other members of the team
Nutrition Therapist
Respiratory Therapists
Pharmacists
Social workers
Coordinators /secretary
Concierges and family liaisons
Chaplains
Therapists: Speech, physical and occupational
Technicians: laboratory, radiology, transportation
Environmental services personnel
Trainees

Chapter 3   Organizing the family
Olivia Brown's family
Organizing your family team
Who do you feel you need around for your support?
Who should be charged with making sure the home and workplace issues are handled properly?
Who has expertise that may help you understand the ICU?
Role of the family in the ICU
Tricky issues with families
Recognize who may become a problem, especially if you are the problem.
Recognize who can be a "hot head".
Enlist other people in the family to help quell family conflicts.
Schedule people who don't get along to visit at different times.
Hospital resources to help deal with family issues
A final note

Chapter 4 Asking questions
The Browns have questions and find their spokesman
Questions: What to Ask of Whom
>I don't know from whom to get information.
>The nurse told me one thing but told my sister something different, whom do I believe?
>When we finally get to meet with the doctor/nurse, I can't remember what to ask.
>Can you please summarize what's going on
>What is the next step?
>What is the long term impact of what's going on?
>I feel there are questions I should be asking but I don't know what they are.
>The doctor/nurse doesn't answer my questions in a way that I can understand.

How does Privacy work in the ICU?
>Who can I contact when I feel I'm not getting the information I need?
>Family meeting and the ombudsman/family liaison office or ethics consultation team.

Chapter 5 'New' Age Considerations
The Browns – it's not all medicine!
Spirituality issues in the today's world
>Religion
>>Non-western methods of healing
>>Bio feedback
>>Relaxation therapy
>>Hypnotism
>>Reiki
>>Feng Shui
>>Acupuncture
>>Making the ICU room a spiritual setting

Resources
Non-traditional families

Chapter 6 Speaking for the Patient
The Browns - Quantity vs. Quality?
End of Life Matters
The patient has talked about what to do if there is a life-threatening situation.
The patient has filled out an advanced directive.
The patient has designated someone to be their durable power of attorney for healthcare.
Accessing the forms.
http://www.uslwr.com/default.asp)
Other End of Life issues
Futility
Do not resuscitate orders and comfort care
Death by Neurological Criteria (a.k.a. Brain Death)

Chapter 7 Organ Donation
The Browns share information about organ donation
About Kristi and organ donations
Making something good from the worst day of your life
Donation after Declaration of Death by Neurological Criteria (DNC) or Brain Death
Donation after Declaration of Death by Cardiac Arrest (DCD)
How do you know if someone wanted to be an organ donor?
What is the process for donation?
for assistance: http://www.uslwr.com/default.asp

Chapter 8 Children in the ICU
The younger Browns have their say

How will the visit affect the child?
How will the visit from the child affect the patient?
Will having children in the ICU be disruptive to other patients or healthcare workers?
Are there realistic risks of children contracting infections in the ICU setting?
Hospital visitation policies
What do you do if the patient is in serious risk of dying?

Chapter 9   Planning ahead
Olivia begins to recover
 Your loved one leaves the ICU
Problem list
Medication list
Looking at your home environment
Picking your doctors
Rehabilitation
Nursing Home
Permanent changes
The challenges of being the caregiver
Losing the sick role
The ICU doctors find there is nothing more they can offer your loved one
Comfort care
Palliative care
Hospice
Preparing yourself
Worksheet 2

Chapter 10   What if --?   Sharing the grief
Your loved one dies
You and your family are going to survive.
There are some administrative tasks that need to be completed.

There needs to be a period of mourning.
A benefit (and comfort) for many families is finding a way to memorialize their loved one.

Decisions to make
Autopsy
Coroner
Giving something back
Grief Counseling

Epilogue   A Happy Ending for the Browns
The Browns a year later

Introduction

As an exercise, some years ago, I asked my secretary to imagine that she was in an intensive care unit (ICU) waiting room; her new husband was admitted to the hospital with a serious illness. I asked her to describe what she would do and whom she would contact. She said immediately that she was wasn't sure. She couldn't think of who in her family to call for help. You see, her mother lives far away, she has friends but is not sure how they would respond to a situation like this. She is recently married and still doesn't feel comfortable calling on her in-laws for help. Luckily, she has no children to worry about.

This exercise was different than the real experience. In the real experience, amid the uncertainty of having someone admitted to the ICU with a disease that is likely unfamiliar to the family, there is the horrible feeling at the pit of your stomach as your mind goes through the multitude of possibilities:

"What if my loved one dies?"

"What if he/she is severely debilitated?"

"What if he/she ends up a 'vegetable'?"

"What if I end up a widow(er)?"

In addition, there are the competing concerns and fears about others in your family group:

"Should the children be involved?"

"Should we call the ex-wife or husband?"

"How to have the in-laws come and visit when you can hardly stand to be in the same room as them?"

As the family member or designated spokesperson, you are being asked to discuss difficult medical issues, make decisions about life-saving procedures, organize family members who are coming to visit, deal with family relationships that may not have been in the best of shape before this emergency, etc. Ultimately, you are also charged with keeping your own sanity so that you can do all the other tasks and prepare for the future. The goal of this book is to help you get through this most difficult time in your life with your sanity and your family intact, and your loved one getting the attention that he/she deserves. As important as that goal is, there are limits to what I can do in a relatively short work. In order to make it readable and useful, I have limited the information. **Specifically, in this book, I will not discuss information about how individual diseases are managed. I encourage you to discuss issues such as these with the medical team treating your loved one.** I fully understand that sometimes communication with the medical team is difficult. Please refer to Chapter Four, titled "Asking questions" for more information about who to contact in that situation.

I have added a *fictional* narrative regarding a family going through the process of being in the ICU. Alex and Olivia Brown are a happy couple who out of the blue are confronted with the hard truth that Olivia is very ill and in the intensive care unit. I will tell you a little bit about their ordeal in the ICU to highlight important issues that will be discussed in the book. The specifics of the illness and their particular family issues are not as important as the way in which Alex, his children, his extended family, the health care team and hospital resource personnel deal with the issues that come up in the ICU. It is our hope that this narrative will make it easier to follow the sometimes complicated relationships and logistics of the intensive care unit.

I start our book with an appendix of common terms encountered in all ICUs. This will help you get familiar with the 'lingo' that all too often healthcare workers use with family members (as though you should understand). Then I will go through the important aspects that you as the family have to address during the critical illness stay, starting from the most critical first day. Specifically, I will discuss how to organize your thoughts and actions in this foreign environment, how to identify important members of the treatment team, where to get information and how to navigate tricky situations where communication breaks down. I will discuss end of life issues that are pertinent for all patients in the ICU not just those at the end of their lives (for example: a living will is for everyone). I will address how to make a plan for the future when your loved one will no longer be in the ICU.

I have tried very hard to make this guide easy to read and informative. I have added two worksheets (see pages 35 and 145) that may be useful to help organize the huge amount of information that you will need to absorb. I hope that during the long hours that are inevitably spent in the ICU waiting room (or in more enlightened ICUs, in the patient's room), this guide will help you organize your thoughts so that the feeling of "not knowing where to start" will not be the defining memory of your experience as a family member of, and an advocate for, a patient who is critically ill.

Take a moment and glance through the table of contents. There is also a list of resources available to anyone anywhere. Naturally, many of the references in this book will be drawn from our own hospital, but most of the information will apply to any hospital and/or intensive care unit. It is not necessary for you to read the entire book from front to back. You should feel free to 'sample' it as you find sections that apply more exactly to your particular situation.

Naturally, I hope your outcome will be a positive one, hopefully on the road to good health and with the hope of being happy again. Unfortunately, not all patients will have the same capability as before their illness, but preparation for the future is a major factor in their recovery.

A Note on Progress in the ICU

Everyone who comes to the situation of having someone in the ICU has different experiences. Maybe you are a healthcare professional or have been a patient in the past. That *can* be a good reference point, however, there is almost no basis for comparison between the hospitals of fifteen years ago and today's medical centers, and most especially the Intensive Care Unit. The management of patients in the intensive care unit has changed almost completely in the 20 years I have been a doctor. This pace of change is certain to accelerate even more in the next 20 years. There will be new technologies to utilize, the machines we use will change, the medicines we use will be supplanted by newer and more effective ones, and there will likely be cures to diseases for which previously we could only offer support.

Specialty ICUs will develop for more and more disease processes that need specific care, and there will hopefully be a major change in the way we approach families in the ICU. I will try to shed light on areas that are likely to change for all patients when that is appropriate. Just remember that even though the machines and medicines will change, the relationships between you and your loved one, you and your family, you and the medical team should remain much the same. I hope this book will therefore outlast the utility of all the textbooks on the shelves in my office.

One important thing that should be mentioned now and will be highlighted later is that there is a push in the United States and Canada to allow family members greater access to patients in order to provide emotional support and, in some cases physical support. Our studies suggest that having families closer to our patients may actually increase their ability to improve. The challenge is to find ways to include families in the room with the patient as frequently and for as long as possible while still providing what are becoming more complicated medical treatments. As we struggle with this concept, we as health care providers have to polish the system knowing that with each new patient we start with novice families. Bear with us. We haven't worked out many of the bugs as yet.

J. Javier Provencio
Kelly Ferjutz

And now -- meet the Browns

Although Olivia has been a loving and careful wife and Mom, always seeing that her family had prompt medical attention when necessary, she tends to downplay such care for herself. She's too busy to be ill, so she just won't consider it. She tends to ignore all the symptoms until it's really impossible to do so any longer, which has previously worked in her favor, as any illness usually disappeared on its own. Generally speaking, she's been healthy for her entire life, and other than when her children were born (easily and quickly) has never been hospitalized. The only doctor she's seen in recent years (on an irregular-regular basis) is her gynecologist. Olivia has never needed a 'primary care' physician.

Now, however, Olivia has picked up the sniffles from her volunteer stint at her son's kindergarten. In spite of various home remedies, she's not been able to shake them, and in the last few weeks, the innocuous sniffles have turned into what she considers to be just a full-fledged cold – although a bad one. In the last week, however, (just when she's the busiest!) she finds it hard to catch her breath at times, and seems to be feverish, off and on.

Of course, this could be part of the 'change' or perhaps just those aggravating hot flashes that are tied to menopause. When a headache persists, followed by dizziness, her husband Alex finally insists that she see a doctor. She resists, claiming she's never needed a 'regular' doctor, nor does she even have one. When she collapses on the floor, and turns weepy (not at all like her) Alex bundles her into the car and heads for the nearest emergency department. It's a completely new world for both of them – not to mention their family.

Alex is astonished to learn that Olivia is very sick, indeed. She has pneumonia, which has weakened her entire body, putting her in a perilous situation. Now what does he do?

Glossary

TYPES OF Intensive Care Units (ICUs)

ICU- Place in the hospital where patients with the most serious illnesses go. ICUs have two important differences from other wards in the hospital: 1) the number of patients a nurse will care for (fewer patients per nurse in ICU): and 2) the type of medications and monitoring equipment available to the patient.

MICU (MRICU) - Medical intensive care is reserved for patients who have problems that do not initially need surgery. These include infections, respiratory problems, and gastrointestinal problems, among others.

SICU- Surgical intensive care unit specializes in patients who have diseases that require surgery, are likely to require surgery, or are complications of previous surgical procedures.

PICU- Pediatric intensive care

Specialty units

CCU- Coronary/Cardiac ICU

NICU- Neurological ICU

TCICU- Thoracic and Cardiac surgery ICU

Trauma ICU- Dealing with patients with injuries from accidents.

Burn ICU-Self explanatory

THINGS YOU FIND IN ICU ROOMS

Endotracheal Tube/Intubation/ "Tubed"- These terms describe the tubes placed through the mouth or nose and into the lung through the vocal cords. This is the conduit by which a ventilator (see below) does its work. In addition to being the straw by which the ventilator works, the tube also allows the nurses and respiratory therapists to suction the lungs, should the lungs make too much mucous. Finally, some patients have a very difficult time coughing up their phlegm (I am sure everyone has had the experience of choking on their own saliva) either because they are too sleepy or because they have problems with their throat muscles. There is a balloon at the end of the tube (imagine a donut stuck around a large straw) that prevents the saliva from going into the lungs. Intubation and "tubed" refer to the process of putting in and keeping in an endotracheal tube.

IV- Short for intravenous catheter and line. These catheters are placed under the skin into the vein to deliver medicines that cannot be given by mouth. They are also good for giving fluids to people quickly if they become dehydrated.

Ventilator- Sometimes called a respirator, this machine provides breaths to patients who can't do it on their own, or may assist the patient as he/she starts breathing on their own. In addition, ventilators can deliver oxygen directly to the lungs in cases where the lungs are damaged and have a hard time getting oxygen into the blood stream where it can be used by the rest of the body.

Central line/Central Venous Catheter (CVC)/Triple Lumen Catheter (TLC) - This is a special type of IV. One of the big limitations of IVs put in the arms or legs is that the veins are small and the skin in the arm tends to become very irritated if the IV is left in for more than a few days. To get past this problem, we have developed techniques to put much larger IV catheters directly into the largest veins near the heart. These catheters can be secured and left in place for longer periods of time without causing irritation. They also have the advantage of making a safer conduit for some medicines that may be toxic if concentrated in a very small vein. Unlike IV lines, central lines are always placed by doctors, physicians assistants or nurses with specialized training. The procedure to put one in looks like a small surgery. These lines also can have complications such as having air leak out around the lung, bleeding or infections. Your doctor or nurse can tell you more about the complications of this procedure should it become necessary.

Arterial catheter - Again, this is another variation on the IV catheter. IVs are placed in the veins (blood vessels that carry blood back to the heart). Arterial lines are placed in the arteries (blood vessels that carry blood to the rest of the body from the heart). The veins have very little pressure. Arteries have the blood pressure that is measured when you go to the doctor's office. A catheter in the artery can directly measure blood pressure continuously without having to blow up a cuff around the arm and listen. For patients in whom the doctors want to keep a close eye on the blood pressure, an arterial line is the favored type of blood pressure device. The arterial line also allows the medical team to do a special test of the oxygen and acidity of the blood without having to poke patients with a needle each time.

DynaMAP/Automated cuff pressure - When close blood pressure monitoring is desired for a patient but in whom continuous monitoring is not necessary, we use an automated system for this purpose. You may notice that you seldom see a nurse with stethoscope in hand measuring blood pressure.

Nasogastric Tube/Feeding Tube - These tubes are usually inserted either into the nose or mouth and go to the stomach where they may be used for more than one purpose. In some patients who may have a problem moving food or stomach juices through the intestines, the tube can be placed on a suction device so that stomach juices don't accumulate and cause the patient to vomit. In addition, medicines you usually take by mouth can be administered down the tube if the patient cannot swallow. Finally, for patients who cannot swallow or can't eat enough to sustain themselves, food (a solution similar to baby formula) can be put directly into the stomach.

Monitor - Although "to monitor" means to watch closely, most people in the ICU refer to the display at the pillow end of the bed that shows heart rhythm and other important numbers as *the* monitor. Nowadays, monitors show much more than they used to. Our monitors can display up to 9 different parameters that include the amount of oxygen in the patient's blood, how fast they breathe, their temperature, heart rhythms, pressure readings from arterial lines and central lines, plus blood pressure. In specialized intensive care units, the monitors can be changed to show very specific information that is important only for patients in that intensive care unit.

TYPES OF TESTS DONE IN THE ICU

EKG/ECG (ECG is the correct term) – An electrocardiogram is an important test that is still used frequently in the ICU. It measures the electrical impulses that cause our hearts to beat. Changes in the ECG can show evidence of heart attacks or changes in the rhythm of the heart. Many newer monitors (see above) can do ECGs without having to hook up any other equipment.

Echocardiogram - (sometimes referred to as 'ECHO'.) An ultrasound test that is similar to the test that is done to determine the sex of babies while women are pregnant. It uses sound waves that bounce around inside the body and bounce back to the machine. The machine then uses these bounced waves to make a picture of the inside of the patient. Instead of looking at a baby, the test looks at the heart. In addition to just putting the probe (and the jelly they apply) on the chest, we have found that sometimes it is better to put the ultrasound probe down the throat into the esophagus (the tube that connects the mouth to the stomach.) This allows us to look at the heart from the inside with a much closer view than is allowed through the chest.

Ultrasound - Exactly the same test described above done for the heart. When it is done to other parts of the body it is simply called ultrasound. The reasons for this name change are largely unintelligible. (Go figure, hospitals sometimes make poor choices). Ultrasound has become a very important technique in the ICU. It used to only be done by radiology technicians, but intensive care doctors have become good at using the technique that has allowed the immediate diagnosis of certain problems and makes it more safe to do certain procedures in the ICU.

Chest X-ray - A long time ago, we realized that for our sickest patients, taking them to the radiology department to get x-rays done was difficult, and sometimes uncomfortable for the patient. Now we have x-ray machines that come right to the patient's bed and take pictures- very convenient.

CT Scan (Computed Tomography Scan- also called a CAT scan) - This is a special type of x-ray. Instead of taking only a single x-ray, a CT scanner takes many pictures, each from a slightly different angle (accomplished by moving the x-ray camera a very small distance before taking each picture). By putting the patient inside a tube that also contains an x-ray machine capable of spinning around (the machine, not the patient!) we get many pictures that encircle the whole body. A computer then uses the x-rays to make a picture of the three dimensional makeup of the body (this is very similar to how phone companies and car makers spin pictures of their products around in advertisements. It is surprising what medicine has done to train people who sell completely different products).

MRI (Magnetic Resonance Imaging) - Despite what most people believe, this is not an x-ray test at all. MRI uses a magnet to make very small changes in the electricity found in all the tissues inside our body. A computer then measures how each of the tissues respond to the change and makes a picture. This is as close to magic as I believe we get in medicine.

Angiogram/Catheterization - This test is a form of x-ray, in which a catheter is placed in a vein or artery and moved to an area of interest. Then, a dye that highlights as bright as bones on an x-ray is injected. Since the dye courses through the blood vessels, the outline of the blood vessels is revealed. This allows us to look at how the blood vessels are working and whether there are blockages. Using this technique, we can also put small instruments into the blood vessels to repair them. The area of interest gives the name to the type of angiogram (heart catheterization, brain catheterization).

THERAPIES FOUND IN ICUs

In this section, I will talk about common therapies you will find in many ICUs. There are thousands of other therapies available to patients based on their needs, but these are the most common. I will also include a few terms that are commonly used in the ICU but will have different meanings than they do in the real world.

Prophylaxis - This is not a single therapy but a set of therapies that we use to protect patients from common side effects to which anyone who is bed-bound is at risk. They include medicines to prevent stomach ulcers; medicines and special boots to prevent blood clots from forming in the veins; interventions done by nurses to prevent the development of bedsores, and sometimes the use of antibiotics around the time of surgery to prevent infection.

Tube feeds - Complete nutrition, high calorie food the consistency of baby formula, which can be given to patients through a feeding tube (see above).

Glucose control - In the last 10 to 15 years, we have become very aware that in patients who are diabetic and in some patients who are not, the level of sugar in the blood goes up in the ICU. This can cause many different problems. We therefore measure blood sugar frequently by pricking a finger or the skin on the arm to get a drop of blood to test. Using this method, we can determine who needs medicine to control sugar and how much.

Blood pressure medicines - many medicines that are commonly referred to as "blood pressure medicines" are used in the intensive care unit to achieve other results. Sometimes these medicines are used for control of blood pressure – whether to raise it or lower it. Also, there are many reasons to use medicines that fall into the category "blood pressure medicines" that have nothing to do with lowering blood pressure. It is common for families to become very worried when they find out that their loved one is on a blood pressure medicine even though they have no history of high blood pressure

Antibiotics - These are medicines that treat bacterial infections. Unfortunately, infections are common, resulting in as many as 50% of the patients taking antibiotics. Limiting the use of antibiotics in the ICU has become a very important issue. It may become important for you as an informed family member to ask the health care team if antibiotics are necessary for your family member.

Restraints - Some of our patients are delirious and agitated due to their illness and medications they receive. If these patients have catheters in place or a breathing tube, they may not be able to resist removing them. We have all had the experience of swiping at a fly that lands on our nose in our sleep while barely noticing what we are doing. The same thing can happen to a patient who has a breathing tube in place. For this reason, we occasionally use soft cloth restraints to prevent this from happening. Because restraints limit our patient's freedoms, there are strict rules that govern who can be restrained and how often doctors need to reevaluate them to see if the restraints are still necessary. Please do not remove or loosen the restraints on your loved one, without first getting permission from the nurse.

Sedation - At times it may be necessary for the health care team to give medicines that make patients drowsy. Occasionally, the patient may need medicines to achieve a near 'coma' condition. This is often times done so that the patient tolerates the breathing machine or during painful procedures. The aim of intensive doctors is to limit the amount of sedating medications as much as possible to prevent complications from the therapy. Sometimes, sedation is necessary for medical reasons that are not directly related to comfort. If you don't understand the purpose of this treatment, ask your nurse.

TWO TERMS TO UNDERSTAND

Intervention - This is a term that is used differently by health care workers and people outside the hospital. In the hospital, we use the term to mean anything we do for our patients that is done the same way every time. This can be anything from putting moisturizing cream on a patient to doing surgery. It means "we are going to do something to the patient." The specific of the "something" is the most important thing.

Procedure - This term is reserved for interventions that are bigger. Usually, something called a procedure will require an informed agreement from the family before the doctor can proceed.

Chapter One
A very bad day for the Browns

Nearing her 45th birthday, Olivia Brown was a typical Midwestern suburban wife and Mom. She did not work outside her home, where she lived with her husband, Alex, and their three kids. Carolyn, 13, is about to enter high school, Alex, Jr. at 11 is in advanced sixth grade classes, and a busy athlete, while Ben, aged 6, will soon be going into second grade. Alex is employed as a purchasing agent for a local manufacturer, and provides well – if not lavishly--for his family. Olivia chauffeured the kids here and there, shopped, and cared for their home, plus, in the last couple of years, has volunteered one day a week in the kindergarten room at her son's elementary school.

Alex is Olivia's second husband: her first marriage was very brief, and her son from that marriage, Tom, is now an adult. Tom lives in a neighboring state, as does his father, and is employed as an EMT, with thoughts of medical school in another year or two. Although Tom doesn't live with the Browns, he is on very good terms with everyone in the family, including Alex.

Once at the hospital, this modest, well-intentioned couple is astonished to learn that Olivia has pneumonia, and she is promptly admitted to the hospital, where care is begun immediately. Within just hours, however, the decision is made to admit Olivia to an Intensive Care Unit, as her condition has continued to deteriorate. Now what happens? Reality can no longer be denied, and the diagnosis/commitment to the ICU has thrown her entire family into disarray.

Alex is faced with taking time off work to care for his children and his wife. At least he does have health care coverage, but he doesn't know if it covers intensive care treatment. He worries:

If she's that ill – to have to be in an ICU – will she survive? What will he do if she doesn't?

Olivia's children are confused and concerned and panicky. What do they do now? What can they do?

Will they be able to visit Mom in the hospital? In the ICU?

Olivia's siblings think their wishes should be considered, too. They want to be involved – she's their sister, after all!

Alex's family is also out there, wanting to be kept informed, and perhaps involved in the trauma that has landed on their family.

When Alex is allowed to see Olivia, even briefly, he is astonished to discover that she is on a ventilator, with a feeding tube in place, and is also sedated. The latter is more for her comfort than any other reason. Alex is desperate to talk to her, to tell her he loves her, and she doesn't respond to anything he says! He doesn't know if she even knows he's there. He wanders blindly through the hallways, finally finding an isolated area where he can sit and weep, quietly. Alex is positive that Olivia is worse than originally thought, and he has no idea how he will cope if she dies. What will he tell the children? How will he care for them while he works?

Voices appear out of his mist, and because of their clothing (dark blue surgical scrubs), he assumes the men are doctors. There are three of them, and as they chat with each other, Alex hears fragments of their conversation. "Mrs. Brown is . . ." but the voice fades. Another says, "Will she last the night, do you think?" while the third one says, "Who could believe this?" And they disappear around the corner (He doesn't realize they are talking about a different patient named Mrs. Brown).

Alex is panicky beyond caring. He *knows* Olivia is dying and no one has told him! They didn't even give him any indication that such a thing might happen. How on earth will he get everyone here – all the out-of-state relatives – in time to say good-bye to her? He just can't lose her! Tears begin to roll down his face, again, as he makes his confused way back to the ICU.

Making sense of the first 12 hours

It is most likely that you have already passed the first 12 hours of your loved one's hospital stay before you picked up this book. In this chapter, the aim is to help make sense of this period and to help you develop a strategy for coping with what is happening. The first 12 hours in the intensive care unit are often times the most crucial of the entire stay. When patients come into the ICU, the process of stabilizing their blood pressure, breathing and any injuries starts immediately. In addition, the process of diagnosing the underlying cause of the patient's instability gets under way quickly.

Typically, when someone comes into the intensive care unit, they have limited or no ability to tell the doctors what happened. As the loved one accompanying the patient, you will likely have been asked a number of questions about what happened (often by more than one doctor or nurse). The questions may include what other medical problems your loved one has, what medicines he/she takes, and any other issues that might have contributed to this illness.

Many family members have told me that about 12 hours later they start having doubts that they have indeed given the doctor all the information he needed. In their heads, they replay over and over the conversations they had with doctors and remember things they forgot to mention (the ankle sprain when he was 15 years old, the history of herpes, the pneumonia she had on their honeymoon).

Rest assured that doctors generally are very skillful in directing questions to family members that will secure specific and necessary information. Without knowing it, you have likely filled in valuable information that was lacking from the information gained from ambulance crews, other healthcare workers, examination of the patient, and previous tests that were done (For example: If you see wires in the area of the chest bone on x-ray, you can guess that the patient had heart surgery). Doctors will come back and ask for extra information if they need it. There are enough other things to think about that you need not worry about holding up your end of the relationship with the doctor. Indeed, at this point, it is essential to move forward with the other tasks you need to accomplish.

The other sentiment that I often hear from families is that the physicians and nurses seem impatient and testy in the first 12 hours. This goes back to the premise that the most important time in the care of most critically ill patients occurs in the first 12 hours. In the beginning of care in the ICU, the medical team must stabilize the patient, figure out what caused the problem in the first place to determine if there are specific treatments to administer, and continue all the care the patient has from previous illnesses.

In the first few hours, doctors and nurses need specific information to accomplish these goals. They use family and loved ones as a resource to reach these early goals. They may appear brusque or short in their attempt to garner the most important data. Do not take this attitude personally. Because of the urgency of that all-important first half-day, doctors and nurses tend to ask very pointed questions that might not make much sense to a family member. This should not be construed as neglect of the family. The medical team needs the benefit of the doubt early in the ICU stay. That will not necessarily be the case later in the stay (see chapter 4 about communication).

Wanting to know prognosis

The first inclination of family early in the ICU stay is to focus on prognosis. Prognosis is the prediction of the eventual outcome of your loved one. However, I can tell you with good certainty that there are very few situations where the prognosis of a patient is clear in the first 12 hours. The most the medical team will likely be able to give you is a series of what ifs (if the blood pressure doesn't respond to medications..., if the infection responds the way it should to antibiotics..., etc.). It is important that the hunt for a prognosis doesn't completely overtake your time and energy. Diseases in the ICU are processes that take time to develop, and may change suddenly and unexpectedly.

In my experience, there have been just as many patients who I thought were going to do well but have unexpected complications that severely alter their prognosis, as there have been patients who I thought were going to do poorly only to make a seemingly miraculous recovery. *Take the information about how your loved one is doing as the most important target of your attention.* If he or she is awake and talking, be thankful that you have the chance to communicate with them. If he or she is not responding to the therapy, use the time to mentally prepare for what may happen. I realize this may seem to put you on an emotional rollercoaster ride, but in my experience, those families who came through the experience in the best condition, always managed to focus on the here and now and believed that a good outcome was possible.

A word about fear. Fear is a very good warning sign of something bad happening. It is important if you are facing a bear in the woods. In a hospital, fear can be paralyzing because so much of what is going on is beyond your experience, knowledge or control. For instance, if your loved one is admitted with a heart attack, fear of his or her dying can make it next to impossible to communicate with your family or with the health-care team. This can lead to fragmentation of opinions, miscommunication with the treating team, and, most importantly, isolation of yourself, at the worst possible time. When people "freak out" in the family room, their loved ones often times don't know how to act toward them so they leave them alone. When someone you love is in the ICU, especially if you are the person helping to make decisions, it is not in your favor to be isolated from the rest of your 'family'. (Keep reading for more on this subject.) You will likely need them at some time in the near future.

The story we always think about is the soldier who is shot but puts it out of his mind in order to complete his task. Although this makes great television, it is not real life. Acknowledging that you have feelings of fear is the first step to controlling them. Trying to put them out of your mind often times causes them to show up in inopportune ways. I had a family member that was so fearful of her spouse dying that she literally couldn't walk into his hospital room. As one would expect, after 20 years of marriage, both the husband and the wife had taken on similar traits. When we finally discussed her fear in the open and gave her appropriate support, she was able to come and visit with him. Interestingly, we were having a difficult time finding out why his heart rate was racing for the first 5 days of his stay. We tried everything to make it slow. After counseling the wife, she went into her husband's room and his heart rate slowed to a normal level. If she hadn't been able to overcome that fear, her husband's care may have been compromised.

Setting up a home base and establishing your 'team'.

The most important thing for you to know and remember, whether you are part of the patient's family or support group, is that you do not need to do everything on your own. Hospitals with intensive care units have enormous resources available to help in almost every conceivable situation. Help IS available; you only need to know how and who to ask for it. In addition to the hospital, you also have family and friends who can lend moral support as well as logistical support if you have to pick up people in the airport, take the kids to school, feed the cats, etc.

The first suggestion I usually make to families is to set up a home base. Find a convenient, specific geographical location in the family lounge, a nearby lounge, or even the cafeteria. This way, any family or friends who come to visit will know where to find you. It will also serve as the first place to look for you when physicians have questions or want to give you an update. Once you have selected the location, be sure to tell the nurse caring for your loved one, and ask for the information to be given not only to all the physicians involved, but also anyone else who may be helping to care for your loved one, such as the social worker or chaplain. It is important for all these people to know, that you can be found at that particular location.

At our hospital, we have an ICU concierge service where an employee is stationed near the ICU to track families and to help them get comfortable. They can be a resource if you don't know where to set up your home base. Other hospitals will give family member beepers so that the nurse and physician teams can find you. This is very helpful. If the hospital has areas that allow cell phone use, it is important to find a space where your cell phone is allowed and has reception. Your support group will have to coordinate between the hospital, the home and work. Having a place where you can use a cell phone without having to run out to the hallway or to the next room can save a lot of time and anguish.

Second, I recommend making a resource list of all the people who can be resources for childcare, home-keeping and work. Matters can become very confusing as one relative after another comes up and asks if there is anything they can do. You may find yourself referring several people to do the same job, while other important tasks are missed. I have heard of one occasion where in the chaos, children were not picked up from school for hours.

When making a list, it should include the resources in the hospital, resources at home, and resources at work. At the end of this chapter, I have included just such a list that you may want to use, and during the course of the book, I will go over all of the categories. You do not need to fill this out all at once. Some of these categories will be easier to fill out over time. The second of these tables is on page 144. I will deal with the first column in Chapter 2, the second column in Chapter 3. The third column, I will deal with somewhat here and readdress in more detail later.

Work issues are easy to forget when the patient first comes into the ICU. Many times, workplaces have resources to help families who have patients in the ICU. In addition, many people have good friends in their workplace. It is sometimes easier to have someone you trust in your immediate family group contact people at work and give them an update from time to time. In some situations, using the information that family members have supplied to their workplace, the workers have been able to fill out all the disability paperwork, present it to the patient's family for signatures and send it through the system. Navigating work disability can be hard for a spouse or loved one who doesn't work at the same place. If co-workers offer to help navigate the paperwork for you – let them do so. This can be invaluable.

There is a great peace of mind in knowing that through all the uncertainty of the ICU stay, your mortgage will be paid and you can continue to buy shoes for your children. Also remember, that if both of you work outside of the house, both workplaces will need this information. In addition, union representatives can be helpful for providing emergency assistance if you need it. There are also resources for the military that can be of help if you, your loved ones or a child is serving in the military. I write many letters for families with relatives stationed abroad for the military to enable them to get leave and come home for a visit.

Limiting Outside Conjecture

The last bit of advice I can offer for the first twelve hours is to limit conjecture. It is likely that you and the doctors have limited knowledge of what is really going on early in the illness. It is often not helpful to have someone making comments such as "my husband was admitted to the ICU and died" or "everyone I know who has been admitted in to the ICU has come out a vegetable". Although these statements may have been true of that one specific instance, it assumes that all patients in the ICU are the same. Believe me, if all the patients I take care of in the ICU died or were left as vegetables, I wouldn't be doing this job. The fact that your loved one is admitted to the ICU suggests that either the doctors do not know the prognosis yet, have yet to discuss the patient's wishes with you, or think there is a chance that they could have a meaningful outcome.

That is not to say that some patients don't end up doing poorly, it just means that some relatives and friends tend to throw out their opinions based on very few facts and very limited experience. Many times, these comments come from their own fears. Admitting the worst scenario is a way of insulating themselves from possible heartache. This may be a good coping mechanism for them, but may be very deleterious to the family group supporting a loved one in the ICU. I realize it is hard to stop some people from saying what they want to say, but it is not inappropriate to take them aside and ask them to be supportive.

It's very natural to become friendly with family members of other patients on the ICU. You are, after all, sharing one of life's most traumatic situations, and this intensity lends itself to reaching out to others who at least know something of what you are enduring. Perhaps they, too, have just come through a similar trauma, or are anticipating one, and fear of the unknown is a great bonding agent. Generally, hospitals do not discourage this attachment, and neither do I.

However, I would caution you about two things. Do not compare illnesses or surgeries between the patients. Each patient reacts differently to the identical illness, surgery and/or medication given, making it impossible for sensible comparisons. Also, it is natural for bittersweet feelings to occur when one patient leaves the ICU before the other does. On the other hand, many long-term friendships have begun in the strange surroundings of the ICU.

HOSPITAL	HOME	WORK
Primary physician:	Primary spokesperson:	Who will contact work:
ICU physician:	Support for me:	Contact person for work:
Other Doctors:	1	Union Rep:
	2	
Primary Nurse:	Family to keep updated:	Patient's contact for work:
Head Nurse:	1	Union Rep:
Social Worker:	2	Military contact:
Chaplain:	3	Disability Rep:
Other hospital persons Job	4	Other persons: Job:
1	5	1
2	Who will care for children:	2
	Daytime:	
3	Nighttime:	3
4	Other:	4
5	Who has medical training:	5
6	1	6
7	2	7
8	3	8

Chapter Two

Alex Brown meets the health care team

Alex is so overwhelmed by the overall hospital situation; he hardly knows which end is up. After his upsetting experience – overhearing bits of conversation about *another patient entirely* – he doesn't know whom he can trust. Of course, he didn't recognize the three men he overheard, and couldn't possibly identify them, except perhaps by the color of their uniforms. But in the ICU where Olivia is there doesn't seem to be any male staff wearing that color.

When he burst into the ICU, panicky, the head nurse intercepted his rush to Olivia's room. A naturally sympathetic person, Mark was ideally suited for his position. He exudes a quiet authority that usually transmits itself readily to those he encounters in his work. He led Alex to a chair, offered him a cup of coffee, and asked how he could be of help.

Alex finally calmed down enough to explain what had just happened, and, while Mark was sympathetic to Alex's fears, he was also able to negate them. Olivia was doing as well as could be expected, and might be taken off the ventilator and have the breathing tube removed in another 24 hours. If she progressed as well as they hoped, she would be on her way to recovery very soon.

As various ICU staff came through the area, Mark intercepted them, and introduced them to Alex, explaining a bit about each person's function on the unit. He carefully stressed that this was a 'team' effort, and thus, it takes the combined efforts of each of him or her to provide the best possible care for each patient. From being confused by the quantity of caregivers tending to Olivia and the rest of the patients in the ICU, Alex was now reassured by their presence, and he began to relax.

It was somewhat calming, and a bit surprising as well, to realize that the various ICU team members were already familiar with Olivia and her illness. The nutritionist was eager to speak with Alex regarding Olivia's favorite foods (not for immediate consumption, to be sure, but possibly with in a day or two) and to inquire about any food allergies. Fortunately for all parties, there were no foods that Olivia could not have, as soon as her system was ready for them.

When the pharmacist stopped by, however, the situation was somewhat different. Alex recalled Olivia complaining about an antibiotic that caused a rash. Unfortunately, Alex was not sure which antibiotic was the culprit, nor the medical reason behind the prescription. Perhaps her gynecologist would know. To Alex's surprise, the pharmacist also suggested checking with the family dentist, and this later proved to be the source of the questionable medication. As it was unlikely that such a medication would be used in a hospital setting, Alex's fears were put to rest.

It was the social worker, however, who provided the most helpful information. When Alex had to admit he didn't have answers to some of Ms. Callahan's questions, it quickly became apparent that he needed help from his family. But which family? He was closer to his own siblings, but obviously they wouldn't be as familiar with his wife's history as her siblings would be. To complicate matters, they didn't all always get along all that well, either. But wait! Her oldest son, Tom, who lived in a neighboring state, was an EMT, and had thoughts of studying medicine. If he could come to be with his mother, he would at least be able to speak the same language as the medical staff, and remove that responsibility from Alex's shoulders.

Having made that decision, Alex immediately felt years younger and his burden became many pounds lighter!

Who is in your health care team – the history

Just as a basketball team has players that do some things well and other things less well, a medical team has practitioners with different skills. Like the basketball team where everyone plays defense but only the point guard is allowed to dribble the ball up the court, there are some functions that everyone participates in and some things that are left to the team members with that special expertise. Knowing who is who in an ICU can be a daunting task. Depending on the hospital you are in, there may be more than one type of doctor or nurse in the ICU with different expertise. Part of the problem with understanding the players in the ICU has to do with two issues that we in the field have yet to fix completely: building the multidisciplinary team and maintaining easy family access to the ICU.

To better understand these two aspects of care, one needs to look at the history of the ICU. Until recent times, the typical ICU team for a patient included a nurse (who took care of two patients), a respiratory therapist if the patient was on a ventilator, and the patient's own doctor (or an assigned doctor if that doctor isn't available). The hierarchy was very clear; the doctor made decisions and wrote orders in the patient's chart and the nurse and respiratory therapist followed those orders.

This system presented two major drawbacks. First, the nurse and respiratory therapist, who had a lot of expertise and worked with intensive patients every day, had no role in the decisions made in the ICU. Second, the doctor who was treating the patient was not a specialist in the ICU and therefore saw fewer ICU patients than the nurses who cared for the patient. This led to other problems; the doctor often made decisions without any input from the rest of the team, or the doctor based his decisions on whatever the nurses said was typically done in the ICU. This system exposed the weaknesses in both the nurses and doctors.

Since the mid-80s, the increasing sophistication of the medical technology and treatments for patients in the ICU has made it almost impossible for physicians not dedicated to ICU care to keep up with the new therapies and machines being brought into the ICU. At that time there was an effort by an already existing specialty group of physicians who called themselves Intensivists (doctors who practice intensive care medicine) to improve patient care in the ICU by standardization of methods and staffing. In other words, to establish the medical professionals as a team, and to operate under team principles. This had many intended and unintended consequences in the ICU. The most beneficial unintended consequence was that the nurses and the respiratory therapists now worked with the same doctors on a day-to-day basis. This allowed much better communications between all the people working in the ICU, and has led to a real team approach for the care of the patient and the family. All the members of the team participate in the decisions but each also has heavier responsibility for their area of expertise.

The one unfortunate unintended consequence of this trend has been alienation of family and primary doctors. Some ICUs have decided to completely disregard the primary physician while the patient is in the ICU (the pendulum swung too far). Our ICU has decided to use the expertise of the primary doctor as part of the team. For who generally knows the patient's medical problems better than the primary doctor?

The second obstacle to understanding the ICU team is the diminishment of the family in the patient's care. In the 80's, when technology, and therefore machines in the room increased, there was an inclination to limit family access. I think part of the reason for this concept was because, in the typical patient's room of that time, there just simply was no room for the family after you put the patient, all the machines and the nurses in the room. In hindsight, this was a mistake. Families who spend very little time in the ICU have a much harder time figuring out what is happening, or who is who on the team, and just what it is that they do. Luckily, there is a very big campaign right now to include families in the care of the patient in a more meaningful way.

I have to include a disclaimer here. This evolution of ICUs has not occurred evenly in all ICUs. There are still hospitals in the United States that do not yet employ an intensive care doctor because the supply of qualified intensive care doctors has not yet met the increasing demand. Additionally, there are still some primary physicians and nurses who believe that the old way is better. The typical arguments are either "Although we never really studied the benefit of the old system, it seemed better," or "I don't need some other doctor telling me how to care for my patients." Feeling as I do that both of these arguments are misguided, I will present only the 'modern' view of the ICU team in the next section.

The care team –

Physicians. In most ICUs there are three teams of doctors. In hospitals with teaching programs, there may also be residents and fellows (doctors who have completed medical school and are in specialized training) attached to each of these teams. This can make the total number of doctors you meet number in the 10s or 20s.

1. The patient's **primary doctor** knows the patient best and decides when the patient needs to go to the ICU. In the best systems, the primary doctor and his/her team remains engaged with the ICU team. They usually meet on a daily basis with the ICU team to discuss the events that occurred overnight. The primary doctor has an important role in communicating with the family, directing the ICU team about events that happened prior to the ICU stay and to help direct medication therapy that will need to continue after the ICU stay.
2. The **Intensivist** spends dedicated time in the ICU. His/her job is only that – ICU care. Intensive care doctors can come from different training backgrounds. Most Intensivists train initially either in internal medicine, surgery or anesthesiology. More recently, neurologists and emergency room doctors are becoming In-

tensivist. Regardless of the initial training, all Intensivists go through specialized training in the treatment of patients with critical illness. A goodly number of medical Intensivists are pulmonary specialists and you may see them in the outpatient clinics. In the best of all worlds, these outpatient duties do not interfere with the time that is spent in the ICU.

The job of the Intensivist is twofold. Because of their special expertise in caring for patients with critical illnesses, they are an important part of the team; generally, they are the leaders of the team. ***The specialty of the Intensivist IS the ICU***. They care for the patient's entire body, not just one organ system or area (as a heart specialist might). As the team leader, they consult with other specialists for help with complicated problems – such as intricate cardiac complications. In that case, the Intensivist will call in a specialist in cardiology to help manage that part of the patient's care. The Intensivists job, as much as anything else, is to be the coordinator of all information including that from consultants. Since consultants narrow their focus to the organ or body system in which they specialize, they sometimes recommend therapies that may contradict another therapy. Knowing which recommendations from the various specialists will most benefit the patient is a major part of the Intensivists job.

Thus, in the core group, the ICU doctor is a sort of clearinghouse for all the information that comes from everybody. The job of the Intensivist is to sort through all the individual reports to be sure there aren't any conflicts. If the nutritionist says the patient has to be fed **right now,** but the surgeon says that the patient is going to the operating room first thing in the morning, a decision needs to be made immediately. You don't necessarily want the patient to have a full belly to go to the OR, as that can increase the possibility of complications. So the Intensivist has to say 'what's the benefit of feeding the patient now versus the benefit of going to surgery in the AM?' That sort of decision-making is

a large part of what we do.
3. The third group of physicians is the **consulting specialists**. Patients in the ICU can have very complicated problems. It is often helpful to have physicians with specific expertise in that particular situation weigh in on the therapeutic options for that problem. There are a number of consulting teams that are commonly called on in the intensive care unit: cardiology, infectious diseases, nephrology (kidney disease), neurology, general surgery, and gastroenterology (digestive problems).

A brief note about **Residents** and **Fellows**. If the hospital you are in has a training program, you may encounter residents and fellows. Residents have already completed four years of college, four years of medical school and may have as many as six years of specialized training (depending on their specialty). Compare this to a lawyer who has four years of college and three years of law school before being qualified to set up a practice, or a pilot for a major airline who has four years of college and a short course in flight school. I always find it strange when patients tell me that they don't want to deal with residents when it is very likely that the resident they are talking about has more education than any police officer, fireman, pilot or congressman they have ever met. I often wonder if this same patient's family members would reject help from a policeman or fireman because they have less than 8-14 years of post-high school education.

Fellows are physicians who have finished their residency but choose to do additional specialization. For instance, my training in intensive care included a residency in internal medicine for three years followed by a two-year fellowship dedicated to just ICU care. That came after the previous eight years of medical training!

The term "intern" is one you may still hear occasionally. In the United States, we don't do rotating internships (rotation between surgery, medicine, obstetrics and pediatrics) any more. We now call our first year residents interns, but technically, they're residents. As residents gain more experience, their expertise improves. It is important to realize that interns are fully credentialed physicians who have a diploma from a medical school that reads "Dr. So-and-So has satisfactorily completed training in medicine and has achieved the rank of Doctor of Medicine" and are always supervised by more experienced specialized physicians.

Nurses. The one constant in ICU care from the inception of ICUs during the polio epidemic of the 1920's and 30's through today's sophisticated care, has been the ICU nurse. Ultimately, the most important intervention offered in the ICU is the close monitoring of the patient which is provided by a nurse. Of all the important changes that have occurred in the intensive care unit over the years with new machines, doctors who specialize in ICU care, and new medicines, this one thing has stayed remarkably the same from the beginning. There should be a close relationship between the ICU nurse and the patient and this happens best if a single nurse takes care of only one or two patients per each shift.

In the ICU, there can be different types of nurses with different training. The majority of nurses in the ICU are registered nurses (RN) who care for patients at the bedside, but there are other nurses as well in an ICU. There are administrators for the nurses in the unit who make schedules and make sure the unit has all the resources it needs to function. These nurses are also the supervisors for the nurses who work in the ICU.

In addition, there are some nurses called licensed practical nurses (LPN) or clinical technicians (CT) in the ICU who are less directly involved in the care of individual patients. Rather, they help the bedside nurses with some tasks like bathing the patient, gathering vital information or making sure supplies are up to date and available for the nurse at the bedside.

Non-physician care practitioners. One of the newer advances to address the ICU physician shortage is to employ Physician Assistants (PAs) and Nurse Practitioners (NPs) who can make many of the decisions physicians make – but under the supervision of an ICU physician.

Other members of the team.

Not all ICUs have access to some of the people mentioned below, but optimally, all ICU teams should have access to all of these services. We have respiratory therapists and a pharmacist who are part of the team and do daily rounds. In addition, we meet once a week for what we call "multidisciplinary rounds" where we invite a nutritionist, a chaplain, a member of the ethics consulting team, a social worker, a speech pathologist, physical therapy, occupational therapy, a position we have in our hospital called the Family Liaison (who is charged with making the family experience more tolerable), our nurse manager and the physicians and nurses who are involved in the care of the patients. At these rounds, we discuss individual patients who may need support from these various services as well as general intensive care unit issues. I will describe how these practitioners are specialized.

1. **Nutrition Therapist**. A nutritionist calculates how much food a patient should get based on the patient's disease, their weight, allergies or other problems they might have, plus other factors, such as foods liked and disliked by the patient, or which might be influenced by religious or ethnic factors. All patients in our ICU have a visit from the nutritionists. We are learning more and more about the importance of good nutrition to patients in the ICU. In some cases, special nutrients can be added to the food to improve the immune system. Since many of our patients are either too sedated or too sick to eat, many of our patients have a tube placed either through the nose or mouth to feed them with a type of food that is similar to baby formula. There are different formulas for different conditions and each patient needs a different number of calories based on the type of illness they have.
2. **Respiratory Therapists** work with patients who have

respiratory – or breathing – problems. This may be as simple as administering the inhaler that a patient uses at home, to managing problems with a ventilator or endotracheal tube. Because so many patients have respiratory problems, respiratory therapists are integral parts of all ICUs. They are also in charge of making sure that the ventilators are in good working order.

3. **Pharmacists** have become ever more important as medicines become more complicated, and there are so many of them. In our ICU, we have a dedicated pharmacist whose job is to make sure that all the medicines we use are effective choices and don't interact with other medicines already being used. In addition, the pharmacist ensures that the dosage is correct and that there is appropriate monitoring of the drug therapy. This is no small task, as many medicines have to be changed depending on whether the kidneys or liver or other body systems are working well. The pharmacist is also the liaison with the pharmacy. There are times in the ICU when we need the medications very quickly, but it is sometimes difficult for the pharmacy to understand 'how quick is *quick*' or who can wait. So the ICU Pharmacist can say "We need *this* medication to come up RIGHT now, but that one can wait 30 minutes or so."

4. **Social workers** can be a very important support staff for families in the ICU. They can facilitate getting work or military leave for loved ones, arranging medications for family members who may have forgotten to pack them, and can help arrange hotel rooms for family members visiting from out of town. In addition, they can be a resource for issues that are not directly related to the patient's current problem.

5. **Coordinators** in almost every ICU serve a secretarial function. They take all the information that is generated in the unit, and put it in a form that can be used for ordering medicines, tests, etc. (This person used to be known as the ward clerk.) Now, almost everything is ordered through the computer, so that job is much big-

ger. They're also in charge of making sure that all the supplies are ordered. This is the person who will likely answer the phone when you call the ICU.
6. Amenities for families in some hospitals include **concierges** and **family liaisons,** whose main function is to help families. Up until recently, it was up to the nurse to handle the patient and family, which often put the nurse in the middle of an ugly conflict. If a family member agitates a patient who is sick, the patient will get worse. It is then the nurse who has to ask the family to change their activity. Having the nurse in charge act as disciplinarian may not be the best thing for the family/nurse relationship.
7. **Chaplains** or on-call chaplain services are present in most hospitals. They represent a man or woman of the cloth who spends time in the hospital. We will discuss this more in chapter 5.
8. **Speech therapist**, **physical therapists** and **occupational therapists** care for the patient's physical needs (especially when they get closer to leaving the ICU). There is a great deal of confusion that is caused by the fact that their professions are named poorly. **Speech therapists**, as their name implies, sometimes work with patients who have speech difficulties. This would seem to be a very small job in the ICU setting. The larger part of their job in the ICU is evaluating swallowing. Many patients in the ICU lose their ability to swallow effectively due to either brain injury, swelling in the throat due to the breathing tube, or because of weight loss that occurs when they are bed-bound for a long time.

Likewise, an **Occupational Therapist** might seem like a strange addition to an ICU team. Job retraining is probably a bit premature in the ICU. It turns out that during the evolution of Physical therapy (which deals with improving strength and balance) and Occupational therapy (which focuses on improving fine motor skills and coordination) different jobs fell to different specialties. In the hospital, this means that **Physical**

therapists concern themselves with big muscle groups usually in the legs and shoulders whereas **Occupational therapists** work with the hands and arms to improve their dexterity. This has the advantage of giving the patient more therapy that we know is good for their recovery.

9. There are a number of specialists who come into the unit but are not assigned to the patients in the unit. These include **laboratory technicians, radiology technicians, transportation specialists, speech pathologists, physical and occupational therapists** that come in and do specific tasks for patients. You can recognize these people by what they have with them. **Laboratory technicians** come to the unit to collect blood samples directly from patients or to pick-up samples. In either case, they usually carry a tray with a handle on the top to hold their supplies or samples. **Radiology technicians** are usually pushing an x-ray machine that looks like a big box with a strange arm coming off of the top. Most people recognize x-ray machines because the end looks like the wall mounted x-ray machine in your dentist's office.

10. The people who keep the whole ICU ship afloat are the **environmental services personnel** who clean rooms and sterilize equipment. (They used to be known as housekeeping or janitorial workers, but they do much more than that.) Often, we take this service for granted but I will tell you that when we have good people doing this function (as we do in our ICU), the infection risk for patients goes down and morale of family and staff improves.

Finally, in hospitals that are associated with medical schools and nursing schools, there are **trainees** who can be in the unit as part of their education. Doctors and nurses always directly supervise these trainees. Even though we think of student learning as a one-way street (knowledge goes into the student), there is good evidence that having students in intensive care units improves care for patients for a number of reasons including improved monitoring of the patients. Also, they're more likely to ask questions, which can be a very good thing, as they sometimes serve in the capacity of 'checks and balances.'

Students can be very difficult to identify, especially if they're older than the typical student. They can look just like doctors and nurses. In most hospitals, students are required to identify themselves as trainees. If you have a question about the level of training of one of the team members, I suggest you ask. Questions like this personally never offend me if they are phrased well. Some physicians may become offended, but that is their problem, not yours.

Chapter Three

The Browns

Alex loves his family. Of course, he does; all of them, even the noisy, sometimes argumentative siblings – both his and Olivia's. He loves his and Olivia's children and even her aged Mom. You could even say he loves Olivia's older son, who is really no firm relation to him. But Tom has matured in the last few years to be the son he'd be proud to claim as his own.

Unfortunately, with Olivia so ill, all Alex wants to do is keep everyone else out, so he can spend all his time with her. Of course, that's not sensible or practical. There is a lot of work involved in being the spouse (or other loved one) of a patient in the ICU. As hard as it is for Alex to do, he'll have to ask for help. And he will, just as soon as he figures out what help is available, and who to ask, and then how to tie the two together.

Tom is an EMT (emergency medical technician) with thoughts of going on to medical school. This makes him the ideal candidate to be the spokesperson for Olivia and Alex. He understands some of the medical language, and even understands the variety of job descriptions of the people caring for his Mom. He can speak their language, then turn around and convey the message to Alex, which makes eminent sense. Except to Alex's siblings. Not being of their family, they think it inappropriate for Tom to have such a position of responsibility, regardless of his excellent qualifications for the task. They choose to ignore the fact that Olivia is HIS Mom!

Alex's oldest sister, Julia, (the only one of his siblings to still live in the same city as he and Olivia) is a secretary for a very litigious-minded legal firm. She is positive that Olivia has not been treated properly, (none of *their* family has ever been in an ICU before now, so why Olivia?) and thinks 'her' attorney can get to the bottom of this strange occurrence. Alex has his hands full trying to convince her to stay out of it.

Then, Julia wonders why on earth Alex has brought Tom in from out-of-state to be the family liaison with the medical team. He's just a boy, really, and after all, she has a college degree! Olivia's brother Jason steps in to confirm that Tom is the best choice. Tom is her first-born son, after all, and while he may be out-ranked by Alex, he's certainly closer to Olivia than anyone else in the family.

At this point, when tempers are really flaring, the parish priest, Father Malone comes in to visit and offer comfort. Father Malone knows Tom very well, and congratulates Alex on his splendid choice of family spokesperson. After all, not every family has such a medically oriented person who can serve in that position. This effectively quiets Julia, and peace reigns – at least temporarily – until she recalls her earlier thoughts of bringing in her attorney employer. Again, Father Malone explains why that is not a good idea at this time. "It's never a good idea to bring attorneys into the equation while the patient is still in the hospital." He goes on to explain about privacy matters and other important considerations, legal and otherwise. He also emphasizes the need for Tom (or Alex) to be readily available in case an important question should arise, and the medical team needs an answer – NOW!!!

Alex is careful, however, to also include Julia in the meeting when he and Tom make up a list of questions to ask the medical team during the family conference scheduled for later in the day. Tom knows to ask the Intensivist to highlight Olivia's condition: highlights as well as lowlights. He then asks what treatment methods are being employed to combat each of the problems, and makes careful notes of everything. In addition, Julia takes notes for herself – in shorthand, proving her importance and usefulness, after all.

Organizing your family team

When you first get into the family waiting room in the ICU, all of your thoughts and energies are directed at the closed doors to the ICU. When you are visiting your loved one, you probably spend all of your time looking at him or her lying in bed. When you are in the family room, you spend all your time thinking about all the possibilities of what might be happening in the ICU. Compounded by the fear of not knowing how this whole ordeal is going to end, it likely feels very isolating. Fortunately, very few loved ones of a patient in the ICU are alone. Usually, there are close family, friends, co-workers and clergy that stop in to wish you well. This is perhaps more common if you live in a small town and go to the only hospital in town.

After a few days in the ICU, the blessings of family can seem more like a curse. It is possible that in some families with adult siblings there are unresolved issues. In today's world of blended families, it may be difficult to cope with an ex-husband (or ex-wife) or the brother you haven't spoken to in seven years.

A few years ago, I treated a forty-something woman patient who developed acute leukemia and had a bone marrow transplant. A week later, she had a hemorrhage into her brain. A week after this when she still wasn't waking up, we realized that she had bled into an enormous lymphoma (a type of solid form of leukemia) that was wrapped around her entire brain.

The time came when, along with her three daughters, we decided that the cancer was too advanced to treat. I asked, "Is there anyone else you want me to notify?" The youngest daughter looked at the oldest and said, "Should we call Dad?" (The parents had been divorced several years earlier.) And the oldest daughter said, "I'll call him in a couple of weeks." My first thought was "That's horrible!" I could never leave a person who was clearly an important part of her life out of the loop for a few weeks. But, it was *their* family, and how their relationships had devolved. This situation occurs quite frequently in the ICU.

How you manage your family and close personal friends can make a large difference in how many resources you can marshal when your loved one needs them most. I find that the most successful families are able to determine how to use their family members to their best advantage. Three questions that may help you navigate this part of the ordeal are:

1. Who do *you* feel you need for your support?
2. Who should be charged with making sure the home and workplace issues are handled properly?
3. Who has expertise that may help you understand the ICU?

Let's look at each of these in turn.

Who do *you* feel you need around for your support?

As the primary decision maker for your loved one (if he or she cannot participate in decisions), you need to remain available so that physicians and nurses can contact you for answers to their questions. It sometimes becomes hard to do simple things such as get lunch or take a nap. Having someone (I will call him or her "the trusted person") who can take some of the burden away can be invaluable. This may at first seem selfish to have someone act as your caddy, but it is often the best thing for the patient. If you cannot function, you cannot make decisions in an intelligent matter. This person may be a sibling, son or daughter, close friend or other relative. It needs to be someone you trust and do not have to be constantly supervising.

My recommendation is to give that person certain responsibilities. Many decision makers will hand over their cell phone to the trusted person so that he/she can screen your calls. If you spend all day answering the phone for every work colleague and well wisher, you will have little extra time.

Another very helpful function of this person is what I call a scribe. Have your trusted person bring a notebook to every meeting with any medical or other personnel and take notes about what is said. I know in my own experience with my parents in the ICU, fear and anticipation interfere with my memory and I remember only about half of what a doctor tells me. Having someone take notes will jar your memory later and may also allow you to think of questions that you couldn't think of "on the spot" during the meeting. Having the trusted person write down questions that come up during the day is also valuable so that when the doctor asks "are there any other questions?" you don't end up blanking and having nothing to ask.

The trusted person can get lunch for you if you want to stay close to the ICU. They can also tell you when it is time for you to go home and get some rest – and you should listen when they do. I personally like it when the trusted person comes to the medical staff and identifies him or herself as such. This way, concerns about the decision maker can be made to both the decision maker and the trusted person. For example, I have had husbands and wives who simply stay at the bedside as long as their loved one is in the ICU. This is immensely draining, to even the most stalwart person. The decision maker can almost never see the effect on himself caused by the sleeplessness and stress they are under. When, as a doctor, I recommend they take a break, sleepless people tend to become suspicious ("why are the doctors trying to get rid of me?"). Having a trusted friend say, "the doctor is right, go get some sleep" can be very helpful.

Who should be charged with making sure the home and workplace issues are handled properly?

Home probably feels a million miles away when you are in the ICU waiting room but bills continue to come, your mail gets delivered, your children need to get to school, you need someone to fill your prescriptions and/or cancel appointments. Designating someone to worry about all these things can be huge relief, but this someone must have a good understanding of your house and your life. Optimally, they will be able to manage your household issues independently, with only occasional questions for you.

Workplace issues are also important. I have seen many difficult situations where someone is in the ICU for a week or two before getting better. At the end of their hospital stay, the family realizes that no one has filed the paperwork for disability or other assistance. This occasionally delays discharge from the hospital while signature pages are sent around to doctors and physical therapists. I mentioned before that when well-wishers from work call (hopefully your trusted person answers the phone) you can enlist them to start the process with these papers early in the hospital stay. They are more likely to understand what forms need to be filled out and where they need to be filed. Work mates are generally very interested – and capable – in contributing to their friend's care by handling these functions.

Who has expertise that may help you understand the ICU?

Some families have people who work in healthcare or who have had significant experiences with ICUs in the past. Sometimes, someone with experience can help you navigate the jargon and help explain some of the medical concepts that are difficult to grasp. Identifying someone with experience and having them on call can be very helpful. This person doesn't even have to be in the hospital. If you have a niece who is a nurse in the next state over, it may be valuable to have her phone number handy. Sometimes, (with the patient's or decision maker's permission) I will call family members who have medical experience to discuss difficult topics. I can discuss the problem or issue using exact but more complicated language and ask the person on the other end how I could best explain it to everyone else. After I get a chance to talk to the decision maker, I encourage them to call their medically savvy family member to make certain there is no confusion about what is being said.

It is important to exercise caution regarding three of

the pitfalls of raising someone up to the position of "expert". First, some people (and we all know them) take the role of expert too seriously and then try to dominate the care decisions. Remember, the decision is still yours to make; the expert is there to advise *you*. Second, some people (and we also know this type, as well) can generalize too much. The classic exclamation I hear is a statement such as "I wouldn't let the doctors start that drug because when I had my wisdom tooth extracted, I had a drug (usually not the same drug in question) and I felt sick for 2 days!" People like this just raise the level of stress for everyone and don't add any special expertise.

Third, some people, when elevated to the level of "expert" can become very condescending toward others. Phrases like "the doctor and I know what is going on, you just trust us that this is best." You will need to fully understand what you are consenting to; and the job of the expert is to sit on your side of the table and explain things in language you understand, not to interject himself or herself as a surrogate doctor.

Not every family has someone with medical knowledge. If that is the situation in your family, often there are resources in the hospital to help. Some patients and families will have a nurse they trust from the ICU sit in all the meetings to explain things. Social workers can also help in this regard. If you have questions about a good choice to be your expert, ask your family members and nurse whom they recommend.

Role of the family in the ICU

It is not uncommon for as many as 20 family members to descend on the ICU for the first few days of the hospital stay. This number usually diminishes as the patient improves or as the stay becomes longer. Many times they have no idea of what they should – or could – be doing. Outside of the few people you have designated to do specific jobs, there seems to be nothing for the family to do. Having said this however, I find that having family around in the ICU is valuable. Sometimes just knowing there is a group nearby that you know and can trust is comforting. This goes for the patient as well. It can be very calming to a patient who is scared – and most of them are – to know the people who are most important to them are nearby. Sometimes families break off into small prayer or meditation groups.

There are a few specific functions that families can perform in the ICU regardless of who they are. Some are very simple. One of the most important of these is to help reduce the risk of infection. There are few absolute truths in the care of patients in the ICU. However, one of them is that we can reduce the risk of infection from patient to patient by **washing our hands regularly**. This is as important for families as it is for doctors and nurses. In a busy ICU, I wash my hands (or use a sanitizer) over a hundred times a day. Despite this, it is easy to forget or get distracted. The family should be the watchdogs for this. If you see a nurse or doctor enter the room and not wash their hands, point it out to them politely. If everyone did this, we could save lives in the ICU. Since we are all on the same team trying to get each patient better, it is reasonable to ask your teammates to do this one simple thing to protect your loved one. I cannot guarantee that every doctor and nurse will be receptive, but I would like to think that most would appreciate a *polite* reminder. Of course, this should be suggested in a calm voice.

A second function that can save lives is to be vigilant about helping to prevent medical errors. It has been well publicized that medical errors account for a significant amount of problems in hospitals and can lead to serious complications for patients. Many mistakes are foolish and simple. They occur because of the number of patients we see and the number of medicines we use. Fortunately, your family only has one patient to worry about. Simple things to look for are: 1) does the name band on your loved one's wrist have his/her name on it and is it spelled correctly? 2) look at any dripping medicine bags and make sure that those also have his/her name on them, 3) keep an up-to-date list of all the medicines your loved one is getting. You don't have to understand what all the medicines do, but just knowing/having the names can be helpful. When a nurse comes in with pills or solutions ask what is in them, or what are they for. If the medicine is not on the list, have the nurse check that it is truly ordered for your loved one. Perhaps the previous treatment has been altered.

Medical care has become very complicated. I think that taking care of a patient in the ICU for a day is probably as difficult as making a car by yourself from scratch every day. In the past, hospitals have excluded family members from helping with the checks and balances. It only makes sense that if you were standing next to someone who was building a car and you noticed that they picked up the incorrect part or a wrong wrench, they should be happy if you pointed that out to them. The same should be true of medicine, but it should be done in a courteous, respectful manner.

Tricky issues with families

I alluded in the past chapters to the baggage that many families bring to the ICU. No family is perfect, and the stress of having a loved one become seriously ill can easily bring out the best or worst of family dynamics. Recognizing that these issues may come up is the most important part of preventing them from distracting you from the job at hand: helping your loved one get better.

Here is a story from my own ICU that demonstrates only too well the difficulties presented by family – and how to overcome and even survive the experience. A patient was admitted with a very large hemorrhage in the back of her brain. She had high blood pressure and was taking medication for it. She and her 'husband' had been together for 26 years, and had a 17 year-old developmentally delayed son. The man worked for the city; however, even though they were not officially married, they were entirely devoted to each other. This woman was dying, and there was nothing we could do for her.

It turns out that the patient had gone out with her sister to a party – a girls' night out. We found cocaine in her system, which apparently is not something she'd ever done before. Her sister all but admitted that she let her try cocaine at this party, and that's probably what precipitated this hemorrhage. The sister had to live with all the guilt. The husband was very angry with his sister-in-law. However, he didn't want to splinter the family so he kept his feelings to himself.

Watching this man find a way to forgive his sister-in-law, rally his family to help, and still care for their child was really interesting – he did a great job. He had his own sister come to help him, while he tried to get his wife's family involved. It was as though these two families were separated by this ugly secret that nobody talked about, but yet no one could ignore. Everyone knew there was a problem – the one sister was beside herself, and couldn't even come to the hospital. He was trying to hold the family together and keep his wife's other sister involved. It was incredibly difficult. He was taking time off work and trying to explain all this to his 17 year-old son who was losing his mother. His family was very supportive of him. Her family tried to be supportive, but they were dealing with an enormous sense of guilt – they were responsible for this situation.

I remember two incidents as if they happened yesterday. The first was the day the developmentally delayed son came to visit his mom. I met with the husband first to discuss how to approach it with him. Then we went out to the family room to get his son. I remember the husband kneeling down on the floor in front of his chair softly speaking to his son (so low that I couldn't hear what he was saying). The child hugged his father and cried. They stayed like this for what felt like an hour.

The other incident was when she finally died. I called the family but had an appointment in the other side of the hospital. I ran into them in the lobby. He sat down in a chair and started to cry (I suspect these two incidents are the only time this man has cried in his entire life). He asked rhetorically "What am I going to do now?" After a moment, he looked at me and said, "I was very lucky to be with her as long as I was. I will just have to move on." It was a horrible situation, but with the help of a very dysfunctional family, he handled it very well.

Too often, family members complain that having their family around is a bigger curse than a blessing. Here are four steps to help minimize the issues around family conflicts:

1. **Recognize who may become a problem, especially if *you* are the problem.**

   The conflicts I see most often in the family dynamic relate to only a few issues that are easily identified. "Entitlement" often leads to clashes between family members. When one family member feels that he/she is more entitled to be part of the family support group, there are always problems. The most unflattering problems occur when the decision maker suffers from this entitlement. This can be as difficult to see in yourself as it is easy to see in other people. I always cringe when the decision maker in the family starts making lists of people who are not allowed to visit. In extremely rare cases, there is good reason to have someone excluded from visitation, but often, it is petty differences.

   When the 'entitled person' is someone else in the family it can disrupt family harmony in the family waiting room as well as the patient's room. Often, this will be a conflict between "blood relatives" and married relatives, particularly in blended families (families where the ICU patient has children from a previous marriage). Some children think that because the new wife or husband has come on the scene lately, he or she should take a back seat in the decision making, even though the new spouse is the *legally*-designated decision maker for the patient.

   Many problems can be settled by taking the people involved to a private place and discussing it before it becomes an issue. If these issues are aired in the family room, you add embarrassment and spectacle to already deep-seated feelings and it can set off a major war of words. If you have the foresight to take the person to a quiet place, you can reaffirm how important all family members are to the loved one's improvement, and discuss clearly how you will be making your decision. For example, "Your father and I have discussed how he would want to be treated if he became very ill. I am going to follow his instructions and make decisions based on what we talked about." In the face of such rationality, even the testiest family members can be won over in the short run.

In my estimation, the most difficult situation for a decision maker is when an ex-wife or ex-husband comes to visit. It's seldom easy to know the right thing to do. In many cases, the former spouse may be the main support person for the patient's children from that first marriage. Providing support may be a vital contribution, but then, how do you say, "Well, okay, come to the hospital but don't see the patient." As in many instances throughout this book, we can only say, "This is our opinion – but there are other ways to do it, too. Each family is unique, and must find the *best* way for them."

2. Recognize who can be a "hot head".

Tensions can flare, especially when there is uncertainty about the outcome of the patient's care. There are long days waiting for any little bit of information. Sometimes the only answers the doctors and nurses can give include "wait and see" and "we aren't sure". This scenario will tax even the most well balanced individual, but some people have difficulty maintaining their cool in this situation. These people tend to blow up, making threats and yelling at whomever they see. This can be an embarrassment for your family. More importantly, it can sabotage your relationship with the doctors and nurses. There are few things that can more easily poison a relationship between a medical team and a family, than constant threats of calls to the administration or instituting lawsuits. They are **totally** counterproductive. In the next chapter, we will discuss further options of what to do if there are legitimate problems with communication between the medical team and the family.

Identifying the person or persons who may sour the relationship with the medical team can be very important. Often, others in the family are able to calm down the hot head. If other family members cannot do this, you may then be left with the difficult decision of asking a family member to leave the hospital for the sake of the patient and the relationship with the medical team.

3. **Enlist other people in the family to help quell family conflicts.**

Often times, there are people who have earned the respect of all family members. These elders of the family can settle disputes in the family simply by asking the participants to stop behaving badly. I have seen many of these elders take a back seat role in deference to the patient's husband or wife. It then becomes incumbent on the husband or wife to give the elder the permission to exert some pressure on the rest of the family.

4. **Schedule people who don't get along to visit at different times.**

There are times when interpersonal relationships between family members are impossible to smooth over. When this happens, it is sometimes more equitable to schedule people who cannot get along. This has to be done with some tact to make sure that one party doesn't feel like he is getting less favorable times than the other. It also means that certain family members may not be invited to the hospital when important decisions are being made. At such times, communication with both parties becomes very important.

Hospital resources to help deal with family issues

There are resources in most hospitals to help families deal with all kinds of issues. If you are having difficulty contacting certain family members, problems getting leave from the military or other profession, difficulty with finances to get family to the hospital, there may be resources available to help you. The service that is most accessible to family is social work. There is a social work office in almost every hospital in the United States. In our hospital, we call on them to work out issues with family or financial issues, as well as follow-up care after the hospital stay.

In addition to social workers, chaplains can be a very good resource for families that have strong faith. Although chaplains usually come from one particular religious persuasion, they are trained in the faiths and beliefs of multiple religions. One should never underestimate the power of a chaplain and family praying together.

You can ask your nurses, doctors or social workers about services available to families. Hospitals are invested in making the experience good, or as helpful as possible under the circumstances, for families. In the hustle and bustle of patient care in the ICU, the family can be overlooked. If you ask for it, there is a good chance you will be helped in a satisfactory way.

A final note

This is how a bad situation can turn out better.
An open letter from a family member in the Plain Dealer (Cleveland, OH) April 26, 2007

"I am extremely thankful for my husband's brothers and sisters and their in-laws for remaining by our side when he was passing away at (the hospital) and all their help afterward with planning the funeral and picking out a cemetery plot. I could not have done it without his loving family."

Chapter Four

The Browns

While listening to Tom blithely spouting all those medical words to doctors and nurses and even other family members, Alex knows he's made the right decision to have Olivia's son be her spokesperson. Of course, even his own siblings still aren't entirely comfortable with his decision, but he is, and they'll just simply have to adjust.

Alex is very impressed with the way Tom takes care to include everyone into the information process. He asked every family member if they had a specific question that he could ask when he met with the doctors. Tom had a notebook in which he wrote questions and comments from everyone, no matter how partial or even trivial they seemed. He told Alex that he'd go through them later to eliminate any duplication before the meeting. The Intensivist had promised a minimum of fifteen minutes –more if his busy schedule would allow – and Tom assured Alex he'd get through the entire list, somehow.

Among the questions Tom keeps on his final list are:

What exactly is her condition now?

Is this different from yesterday or the day before?

Is this likely to change by tomorrow, for better or worse?

What is the best treatment for this condition?

Does she need to be seen by any particular kind of specialist?

What are the problems to overcome right now?

What is the next step in her care - the next decision?

Is there a long-term impact on what is happening?

If there is more than one condition, what is the best treatment for each?

Please summarize what is going on? What do I

need to know?

    The meeting with the doctor, Alex, Tom and Julia went well. Alex is pleasantly surprised when Tom and Julia emerge from the consultation smiling and talking together. It seems she now approves of Tom very highly. Indeed she sings his praises to anyone who'll listen! "He was so calm and collected, and very polite to the doctor, who responded accordingly." Somewhat abashed, she continued, "I couldn't have done as well. Tom was so knowledgeable and respectful." High praise indeed!

    Generally, nothing is for sure, but the Intensivist foresaw no immediate changes in Olivia's condition, and expected her to make a good recovery, if not necessarily a speedy one. "These things all take time," he assured Tom and Julia. At some point, she would be able to leave the ICU for a medical floor, where she would probably stay for another week. They must be sure she was able to care for herself and her family before she could be released. Usually, pneumonia was not a long-lasting illness, once treatment was begun. None of the tests so far indicated the presence of any other condition, so at this point the outlook and prognosis was positive.

    It was a very happy family gathering that night, especially as Julia continued to be lavish in her praise of Tom's demeanor. Alex could literally feel the bonding between the two sides of his family. He began to hope. . .

Questions: What to Ask of Whom

The questions that all families invariably ask me after their loved one has been admitted to the ICU revolve around other *questions*. Typically, there are five different areas of concern that occur – each with its own set of questions and answers. In addition, we will talk about privacy issues in the ICU and what happens when communication between the family and health care team breaks down.

The five areas of concern about which families come to me for help are:
 1. I don't know from whom to get information.
 2. The nurse told me one thing but told my sister something different, whom do I believe?
 3. When we finally get to meet with the doctor/nurse, I can't remember what to ask.
 4. I feel there are questions I should be asking but I don't know what they are.
 5. The doctor/nurse doesn't answer my questions in a way that I can understand.

Not long ago, the daughter of one of our patients started yelling at the top of her lungs that she was going to sue everyone in the building. I was called in to calm the situation because I had a good relationship with her. When I sat down with her in a quiet room and asked why she was so upset, she said no one was caring for her mother. I asked what she meant by that and her response was surprising to me. "I don't know why I think that, I just do." I asked her if I could answer any questions for her and she started to cry. She said, "I don't know what to ask."

We started at the beginning with why her mother was in the ICU. I felt rather silly starting with information that I felt we had been over many times before. I thought she would think I was talking down to her. She stopped me after a few sentences and said, "I didn't know she needed a machine to keep her breathing." It occurred to me that she had never asked why there was a big tube sticking out of her mother's mouth that was attached to the big machine in the room. I just assumed the big machine was self-explanatory. Often, patients' families, in the stress of the situation don't catch obvious facts.

This woman was an administrator in a well-respected government office. I am sure she could pick out the brand, year and paper type of any printer in my unit. Yet as a daughter, when her mother was sick and she was stressed, she missed the 300 lb. machine making huffing sounds in the room. She didn't know what questions to ask because she was too overwhelmed to identify the important clues that were clearly visible. This left her feeling frustrated. After a good discussion of all of her mother's problems, the daughter was calm and happy with her mother's care. In my experience, when families are frustrated, more communication can only improve the situation.

1. I don't know from whom to get information.
This can be a daunting task. Most family members want to talk to the doctor frequently but if a doctor meets with the family of every patient for an hour a day and, as in my unit, the doctor takes care of between 16 and 18 patients . . . well, you do the math. This is in stark contrast to the family's perspective. Because to the family, this is likely the most important time in their loved one's life, they don't really care about what the doctor's schedule looks like. How would you feel if you were in a burning building and the fireman said "you are going to have to wait because I am really busy just now"? This tug of war between the doctor's reality and the family's reality is frequently a source of tension. Negotiating this conflict can take some delicacy on both sides.

There are a few steps that family members can take to help manage this issue. The subject of who to speak with, and what to speak with them about, will be discussed again later in this chapter. First, get as much information as you can about your loved one from the nurse. It's easier to identify the nurses than others on the team, because in most ICUs the nurses are assigned to only one or two patients.

Although they are very busy, they can often talk while performing other tasks. Throughout the day, a family can frequently talk to a nurse if need be. This can limit the time you need to spend with the doctor.

If your ICU uses the team approach, the nurse will have participated in daily rounds with the ICU team, which includes the doctor. The nurse should know what was discussed at the rounds and should have a clear update from the previous shift nurse regarding the patient's experience during the last 24 hours. In many cases the nurses know as much about specific patients as the doctors. For example, if a patient needs a water pill to decrease swelling but has never been on the medicine before, it is difficult to predict the correct dosage. On rounds, the ICU team may decide to begin with a small dose to see how the patient responds. Usually, they establish specific parameters such as: if the patient doesn't urinate a certain amount by a specified time, the nurse is to give a second dose of the water pill. If the doctor is busy dealing with other issues, the nurse may have the information about whether the medicine worked and what subsequent doses were administered long before the doctor has the information.

The nurse can also be a valuable resource to explain the medicines and equipment being used in your loved one's care. Just like the woman mentioned earlier who failed to notice the ventilator, it is easy to miss things in situations as complicated as an ICU. I find that families that ask the nurse "What are all the machines and what do they do?" or "What are the medicines hanging from the IV pole?" and "What medicines are you giving the patient and what do they do?" have a pretty good understanding of the care that is being administered. This will also serve as a springboard for questions about why those specific treatments were chosen. Finally, it may help craft additional questions to ask the doctor.

Once you have gotten information from the nurse, it is important to have contact with the physicians. The question of which physician to talk to can be tricky. The primary care doctor will have a broad idea of what is going on with the patient and how it may impact the patient's long-term survival but he/she won't have a good grasp of each medication and every detail of the care. Some families like to meet with each of the consulting physicians involved in the care. However, this can be very confusing.

For example, if the patient has a bleeding ulcer, the ICU team may call in the gastroenterologists (GI doctor) to consult. Depending on the patient's general health, certain options may not be available. If the family asks, "What is the best therapy for the ulcer?" the consultant will likely tell you that surgery or a camera procedure is the best therapy. Unfortunately, if the patient is too sick to tolerate the procedure, the intensive care team may have to use other, lesser options. The consultant may not know all the extenuating circumstances until after meeting with the ICU team. This can then confuse family members when they find out their loved one is not getting the 'best' treatment as outlined by the consultant. I find it best for the ICU team or the primary care physician to recommend when family should meet with a consulting physician.

The best types of family interactions with doctors come when the ICU physician and primary doctor can meet together with the family. This way, the person who knows the details of the care (the ICU doctor) and the doctor who knows the longer-term course (the primary doctor) are right there in the room together. If scheduling of this is problematic, then the safest person for the family to meet with is the ICU physician.

2. The nurse told me one thing but told my sister something different, whom do I believe?

This is a very common problem. When you think about the stress you are under, it is difficult to understand all the information that is coming at you. As an example, my father (JP) was in the ICU after cardiac surgery 3 years ago. As the physician in the family, I was the person who met with the doctors. I was amazed that through the haze of anxiety about whether my father was going to be OK, I could remember only about half of what the doctor told me when I went back to report to the rest of my family. And, I had the advantage of understanding all the words and being familiar with the ICU setting (although it was a different hospital). I suspect that less than half of the information I discuss with a patient's family is remembered. So, many times, the problem is that the information getting back to the family is not complete.

Everyone played the game of telephone as a child where one person would whisper something to a person next to them who would do the same until it comes back to the original person. The point of this game is to see how different the story becomes with retelling. This happens with our patients as well. It is common that I will tell the exact same thing to two different family members and later find that they each have a different understanding of the conversation. Also commonly, I find that two family members will be told different versions of the same story and then regroup. When they put the story back together between the two of them, it comes out very different from the original. This situation creates very confused and unhappy family members, which can easily interfere with the patient's well-being and recovery.

To counteract these two problems (the haze of anxiety and the 'telephone problem'), I suggest that early on in the ICU care the family designate one person to be the **Contact Person**. This person doesn't need to be the decision maker. The qualities you need in the contact person should include clear-headedness in difficult situations, reliability to ask questions that are brought up by the family, *good note-taking skills* (and the presence of mind to always have handy a notebook of some sort plus a reliable pen), and the ability to learn new concepts. Having medical experience or knowledge is helpful sometimes, but can also be a problem. I know personally, the hardest family members to deal with are those who have some medical knowledge and try to generalize all the information they get (i.e. "I saw a patient in the nursing home who looked really sick until they started antibiotics, then they improved a great deal. Maybe Mommy needs antibiotics." This comment was about a patient who had no infection and looked sick because of her major stroke). The job of the contact person is to gather the thoughts of the whole family before meeting with the ICU team, make sure all questions are answered, and then report back to the family. Although this system of a contact person still leaves the problem of not remembering well, a contact person who understands his/her job is more likely to remember more.

There are a few added benefits to having a contact person. Patients in the ICU can have rapid and profound changes in their condition. Sometimes when those events happen, procedures are needed to stabilize the patient. Having a contact person gives the nurses and doctors one phone call to make or person to find in the hospital with whom we can discuss these issues. The contact person can then call all the other family members and mobilize them. This also makes it easier for the doctors to discuss procedures that need to be done and the risks and benefits in the event that the patient cannot consent for himself or herself.

3. When we finally get to meet with the doctor/nurse, I can't remember what to ask.

It is often difficult to think of questions to ask when you are standing in front of the doctor or nurse. It is common for a patient's family member to tell me "I had a lot of good questions in the family room but now I can't remember what they are." There are a few good ways to get past this problem. We've already mentioned one such method; write down your questions as they come up. (It's a good idea to always use the same notebook for this purpose, even if your scribe changes throughout the ICU stay. This aids continuity.) Another strategy is to have a series of questions you can fall back on, if you get stuck, that will likely give you all the information you need. Here are a few suggestions.

One good question family members can ask is **"Can you please summarize what's going on?"** Once you have that information it may jar your memory for the question you intended to ask, generating new questions or simply answering your question before you need to ask it.

The reason that this one question is so powerful can best be illustrated by an example. Someone with **sepsis** (profound low blood pressure due to infection) in the ICU has a number of things going on. As far as therapies go, we initially start antibiotics to treat the infection. We give the patient medicines and a lot of fluids to get the blood pressure up. Maybe the patient is on a breathing machine. In addition, we often start medicines that will protect the patient from problems such as blood clots in the legs and ulcers in the stomach. Finally, the patient likely will continue on the medicines that treat all the other problems they have at home. So for the doctor to describe all of these things is difficult. You can focus the doctor on what he/she should be telling you by asking the question: **"Please summarize what's going on?"**

A good second general question to ask is **"What is the next step?"** Although it is important to get information about what has gone on and what the situation currently is, it is just as important to know what may come next. If there are decisions to be made in the near future – such as: decisions regarding possible treatment options or patient's wishes – it is better to have a lead time to discuss the decisions with other family members than to have to make decisions quickly when there is no time for contemplation. A good example of this from my experience in the medical ICU is the patient with severe emphysema who has pneumonia.

Initially, the ICU team may try to support the patient with extra oxygen and medications. If the patient doesn't respond, a breathing tube and breathing machine may be necessary. In the initial discussion with the doctor, if the question about the next step is discussed, the family will understand that the next step may include placing a breathing tube. This may remind the family about discussions the patient has had about being on a breathing tube, which could open up conversation about other options. If the possibility of placing a breathing tube is never discussed, the decision about whether it is the right thing based on the patient's wishes is pushed to the time when there is no time for discussion. You can imagine how differently these two conversations could be and how they might affect the patient's care.

The third question I find helpful is **"What is the long term impact of what's going on?"** This is best described with two examples. Looking back to the example of the patient with sepsis (infection and low blood pressure) and another example of a patient with a large stroke is helpful. Obviously things can get worse over time in the ICU if there are complications, but the patient who has sepsis (although at high risk for dying in the ICU) has a good chance of getting back to their normal life if he/she survives. Someone who has a stroke in their brain has a lower likelihood of dying in the ICU, but, even if we can get him or her through the ICU stay, he or she is likely going to be weak on one side the rest of their life. There is a good chance they will not be able to go back to work again. So in the planning stages early on, you can get some idea of how to plan your future.

4. I feel there are questions I should be asking but I don't know what they are.

This is a common fear. The nurses and doctors should make sure you have a good working knowledge of what medical facts are important. If they don't, the questions above will give them a reminder to explain everything. Some family members ask friends or relatives with more medical knowledge to sit in on meetings with the doctors and nurses to ask questions that may seem inappropriate or embarrassing. If you don't have a relative or friend, you can ask a social worker, family liaison, or chaplain to do this for you. However, non-medical personnel may have less medical knowledge than the doctors and nurses, which means they might not catch if someone slips in a piece of medical jargon. Ultimately, it is your responsibility to ask questions until you understand what the doctor is saying.

A quick note about TV dramas; as a way of making actors playing doctors sound more credible, they often say things to families such as "Because your mom went into V-tach, we had to do an ABG, EKG and a 2D Echo." Unfortunately, the younger generations of doctors in training who apparently watch these shows seem to think this type of abbreviated mish-mash makes them sound more professional. I wish people in our profession would read about the real superstars of medicine of the past 100 years who understood that you speak to families respectfully and at their level of understanding. This reminds me of a quote by Albert Einstein when he was asked how he could tell if someone was intelligent. He said, "A sure sign of intelligence is when a speaker speaks at the level of his audience." I urge all of you to not let doctors get away with sloppy speech. Call them on it and have them explain it to you in a way that you can understand.

One way of making sure you are getting all the information is to ask the doctors to go through everything systematically. In the ICU, patient problems get complicated very quickly. In the example of the patient with sepsis, not only do we have to worry about the infection, we also have to worry about the blood pressure (cardiovascular system), the lungs (respiratory system), ulcers developing in the stomach (GI system), effects of the infection on blood cells (the blood system) and so on. In addition, these problem often lead to others; for example, if our patient has respiratory problems requiring a breathing machine, they will likely need sedative medicines to help them cooperate with the machine. Now the brain is involved.

In order to tackle all of these issues and keep everything straight so we don't miss anything, we usually make up a problem list for each patient. This is done either by logging all of the patient's problems (cannot breath on their own, cannot get out of bed, cannot eat, etc.) or by going through a list of body systems and determining whether that system is affected (kidneys, liver, lungs, etc.). The point of this exercise is to make it easier to understand what is going on in a very complex system. You can use this to your advantage by asking your nurse or doctor to go through a list of your loved one's problems and how he/she is being treated for each of them.

I will warn you that even for a patient who is going to do well, the problem list can get very long. The main reason I worry about recommending this strategy is that some families become fixed on every little problem. There are times when for the greater good of the patient, we recognize problems but don't treat them. This can be difficult for a family member to understand. The best example of this is a patient I had in the ICU recently.

The patient hadn't been fed for two days, because he had developed inflammation of the pancreas. The treatment of pancreatitis includes stopping feedings until the inflammation begins to resolve. So the patient had two problems on the list that contradicted each other. We couldn't feed him because of the pancreatitis so one his other problem, not being fed, was not addressed. The family was very uncomfortable with this and asked us to try to find some other way of feeding the patient. There is an intravenous feeding solution, which can be put directly into the veins. We entertained this, but this solution can make infections worse which is why we couldn't use it. So you see, one problem (feeding) interacted with two other problems. Although this may be a good tool to understand medical data, it can be hard to comprehend the big picture if you get caught up in too many details.

The risk of focusing so hard on the details for a family is that you miss the forest from the trees. I have seen families become completely infuriated because their loved one has low blood counts and completely ignore that the patient has a stroke that is not survivable. By focus on the details, some family members insulate themselves from the hard truths that they don't want to confront.

5. The doctor/nurse doesn't answer my questions in a way that I can understand.

This is the source of the most frustration for a patient's family. Anyone, including your doctor or nurse can have a bad day or a personality clash with a family. I have had some families that have been very difficult for me to connect with for reasons that were not anyone's fault. It is the job of the nurse or the doctor to find some way to remedy this situation. Two avenues that are very helpful are the **family meeting** and the **ombudsman's office or ethics consultation team**.

Many doctors in the ICU meet with families at the bedside informally during the day. This is convenient because you don't have to plan a meeting and as the doctor walks about the unit, he/she steps into the patient's room, gives a quick update to the family and then goes on about their business. During a typical day, you tend to get to every family for an update. Occasionally, you miss the same family over and over again. This can lead to confusion and alienation on the part of the family. What I suggest is that the family asks for a **family meeting**. This is a scheduled meeting with the ICU team to go over the care of your loved one. It sets a time on your doctor's schedule when you know you are going to have time to discuss your concerns. I have found that this type of meeting usually resolves many issues and resets the relationship between the family and the ICU team.

The family meeting should be in a quiet place where you can be seated. Some hospitals don't have rooms available all the time so you may have to be flexible. I would also recommend having as many interested family members and friends attend as possible. This will allow them to hear directly from the doctor what is going on. It is also helpful if the nurse at the bedside can join the conversation to complete the picture.

When the family meeting starts, I find it helpful when families ask how much time I have to discuss things. There are days when I have 5 family meetings scheduled in half hour successions. If your doctor tells you he/she has no other commitments, you can sit and chat about anything you want. If the doctor has only 15 or 20 minutes, you may want to get to the important questions right away. It is helpful if one person asks the questions. This eliminates the problem of five different family members asking dueling questions. At the end of the meeting, I usually ask other family members if they have any unanswered questions. This provides everyone a time to be heard.

Many times, doctors and nurses will initiate a family meeting if there are decisions that need to be made and the patient is unable to participate in the discussion. These meetings are very important and are not usually called lightly. If you hear that the ICU team wants to have a family meeting, you should find a way to make yourself available.

If you try to initiate a family meeting and it doesn't go well or if you cannot get the doctor or nurse to commit to a meeting, there are other means. Every hospital has a mechanism for families to raise grievances while in the hospital. In our hospital, we have an **ombudsman's office** (a fancy word for a liaison with families). Although they dutifully document complaints from families, in our hospital they do much more. They are an effective group of people who have the support of the hospital administration to fix problems. They usually do this amicably and without blaming the doctor/nurse or family. I find them so useful that if I notice that the relationship with a particular family is not going well, I will often call them to come and consult. I had a family member ask me if that amounted to me "telling on myself" but I don't see it that way. My goal in the ICU is to try to improve the life of the patient. The family has the same goal so we are really on the same team. If we are not communicating well, then the team suffers. Asking a coach to come and help fix the team makes sense.

If the problem with the nurse or doctor has to do directly with the care of your loved one, there is an **ethics committee** or service in every hospital designed to look at these issues impartially. You can ask your doctor or nurse to consult Ethics. If the doctor or nurse is unwilling to do this, many hospitals will allow families and patients to consult them directly. The ombudsman's office can help you with this.

A final word about conflicts with the ICU staff; I have never seen a family get any benefit from getting a lawyer to try to mediate or threaten doctors or nurses while the patient was in the hospital. This may seem self-serving on my part to say this but I assure you it isn't. Any lawyer worth his/her salt won't come into a hospital while a patient is still critically ill and start threatening lawsuits to try to get the care to change. In today's society, it is very tempting to tell doctors "I will sue you" but, in reality, families who say those things don't usually sue, either because they don't have a case or because it is said in haste. If you feel that there is malpractice in the care of your loved one, it is appropriate to get a lawyer involved during the hospital stay and to move your family member to another hospital if you feel their care jeopardizes their safety. But to have a lawyer confront a doctor or nurse in the hospital without access to all the facts (the patient record isn't completely compiled until the patient is discharged from the hospital) is folly.

How does *Privacy* work in the ICU?

Patient privacy – or privacy of information is a very big problem in the hospital. No one wants to think that personal information about health care issues is being broadcast to everyone in earshot. Having said this, information in the ICU has to be transmitted quickly in order to make decisions that impact patients. Over the years, doctors and nurses had lost some of the sensitivity about personal information. We felt that nobody really cared what was said, (or wouldn't understand it) and people would walk around the hospital talking about Miss Jones who had this procedure or hepatitis, not really appreciating that this information might be considered private by patients and their families. We forgot that the personal and healthcare issues that patients entrust us with are secrets that we don't have the right to disseminate. The government is now very interested in the concept of privacy for the patient, as are hospitals.

Psychiatric wards have always been careful about their records, but the general hospital community decided we had to be more careful with everyone's records. Interestingly, it was the AIDS epidemic that really changed everything. Having a disease that was considered taboo changed our thinking about privacy issues in regular hospital wards. In large part, this was to protect those people who had HIV (or a related illness) and thus have problems with their jobs or their homes if such information became public.

What this means for you as a family member is that you shouldn't hear about other patients when you're in the ICU, nor should you expect others to hear about your patient, either. Although we can't control the curiosity of patient's families, we expect visitors in our unit to focus their attention on their own loved one and not on what is going on with other patients. That is not to say that you cannot strike up a friendship with some other family and discuss the specifics of their healthcare problem. As long as the family volunteers the information, this is fine. We expect that as visitors in the unit, you will not ask our nurses or doctors private information about other patients. Although this seems obvious, it is not always so. It is very tempting when you see a patient being wheeled through the hallway, to innocently ask the nurse in the room "What is wrong with that person?" The nurse should stop and politely tell you that he/she cannot talk about it.

Of course, this also means that doctors and nurses are very limited as to whom they may give information. So every patient's family member should carry information as to who is next of kin – or a spokesperson. If the family designates a spokesperson, regardless of whether that person is a next of kin or not, then the physician will speak to that person only – the one identified by the family. Otherwise, only the family will get information. If the pastor calls, he's not going to get any information. If an interested friend calls – even if the interested friend is a medical professional, we can't give them any information.

It's very important for people to know that while we safeguard information about patients, it also means that very interested, very loving friends and/or family will not be able to receive answers. Even if they've known the patient for forty years – the nurse basically has to say, "I'm unable to give you that information. I cannot tell you anything." It's not that we don't want to share information it's that *we can't*. That's for the protection of the patient.

The nurse may ask, "How are you related to the patient?" Sometimes friends come or call and get very angry because they can't find out how the patient is doing. "I just wanted to know how he's doing" and we can't tell them. So we refer them back to the family, preferably the family spokesperson. It's good when we can give them a name and a phone number, and that person can then provide whatever information should be given out. We like to be able to say, "The only person we can legally tell is *(name of family spokesperson)*. You can contact them at this number."

Chapter Five

The Browns

Now that Olivia was responding to treatment and seemed well on the way to recovery, tensions in the family grouping lessened considerably. There was still the occasional flare-up as when her sister Marcia suddenly asked if anyone had requested the Last Rites to be read over Olivia. As Alex's family was not Catholic, this caused a few heated words, before someone suggested asking the hospital chaplain for advice. Father Malone was once again called upon for advice and counsel, and to Alex's surprise, the priest states that Last Rites may be read any number of times for the same patient, and not infrequently, it is of more comfort to the family than the patient. Alex agrees to Marcia's request, and the family gathers around Olivia's bedside for the occasion.

Later that evening, Father Malone again appeared in the ICU, but in a more somber mood than he had been earlier. Marcia started to call out to him, then, realized he was going to the room of a patient down the hall. She stood quietly, watching, and suddenly started to cry. Her husband Blair, surprised at her emotion, asked what was wrong. "I think that Mary's husband must have died." Mary and Marcia, who are similar in age met in the waiting room and the two women had chatted frequently during Olivia's stay in the ICU.

"Why do you think that?" he asked.

"They brought up a gurney, and after Father Malone came up, they closed the door to the room. They *never* do that!" That was true. ICUs tend to be very open, for the sake of both expediency and convenience. "Oh, dear. Poor Mary," Marcia sighed and turned into Blair's embrace. "I'll really miss her," she said looking up at her husband's face, before tears struck again. "I wonder if I should go to her?" she asked of no one in particular.

"I think you should stay here," Blair answered. "If Mary wants you, she'll know where to find you." Guiding her with his arm around her, they walked to the other side of Olivia's room. Marcia still shed tears occasionally throughout the next few hours, as she thought about her new friend.

Later that evening, when it seemed that once again Olivia was resting somewhat more peacefully, the family began chatting quietly among themselves, at the far end of Olivia's room. Olivia's brother Jason wonders aloud about some of the 'new age' topics he's heard being discussed at work and at church groups. Among these are Bio Feedback, relaxation and hypnotism. Nearly everyone there has a story about someone they know who benefitted from the 'treatment' but in every case, the patient was able to participate actively in the routines. Since Olivia is not yet that far advanced, they pass on those topics.

Julia, being more aware than most offers up her admittedly scattered knowledge of Reiki and Feng Shui. She's not participated in them herself, but 'knows someone' who has, with great success. Again, however, as Olivia is still bed-bound and liable to be so for some days, it seems unreasonable to pursue either of these ideas.

"Ah! But what about acupuncture?" asks Alex's brother, Henry. Everyone in the room cringes slightly at the thought of yet more needles. But, again, it seems that each of them knows of someone who was helped by this admittedly exotic form of treatment.

Just then, Mark, Olivia's main nurse enters the room. Before he can say anything other than 'hello,' he is bombarded with questions about this method of treating illness. Displaying his usual patience, he carefully – but briefly – explains why Acupuncture is seldom allowed in the ICU because of the high risk of infection, which is already high in the confined area of the ICU. However, that is not what brought him here. He really came to speak – rather urgently, in fact – to Alex and Tom, with some difficult questions.

"Mr. Brown, we're still having some difficulty with your wife. Mrs. Brown is not doing as well as we'd hoped for." The nurse was not smiling, as he had in the past.

"Is she – ?" Alex stopped speaking as his throat closed. He felt Tom's hand on his shoulder, offering comfort.

"Does my Mom need surgery?" Tom asked.

"We're not entirely certain. Her vital signs have just gone berserk again, and we're doing our best to get her stabilized. But, just in case, if there's anyone you'd like to notify, this might be a good time to do so."

Julia interrupted. "Just what do you mean by berserk? Can you explain that a bit better?"

"She may be having a heart attack. Her blood pressure dropped very suddenly, and she's in respiratory distress. We've increased her oxygen, but it isn't helping so far. There are some hard questions we have to ask of you."

"Should we call Father Malone?" asked Tom.

"Certainly you can if you want to. But first, do you know if Mrs. Brown has ever filled out any kind of medical advanced directive forms?"

"Do you mean a living will or something like that?" Tom looked at his step-father, confusion on his face.

Alex could only shrug his shoulders. "I don't think she's done any kind of will, living or otherwise."

"Is she dying? Is that what he's trying to tell us?" asked Julia, bursting into tears.

Spirituality issues in the New Age

Faith is a very personal – and individual – matter, and the comfort it can provide should never be underestimated. Many families and patients I talk to tell me that they made it through the tough times in their hospital stay because of their Faith. It is also true that when people of different religious beliefs or no religious beliefs are scared about the outcome of their loved one's illness, tensions can arise based on whether someone has the '*appropriate*' faith. Regardless of whether it is the patient or the family who derives the most benefit from Faith, it is very important to be sensitive to other people's beliefs. This can be especially crucial if family and friends are of different faiths.

The issues of Spirituality or Faith include many topics of a much broader nature. We will cover some of these issues that are important for patients and families. They include:
1) Issues pertaining to organized religion
2) Non-western forms of healing
3) Making the ICU room a spiritual environment
4) Resources for families

As a quick disclaimer, I am not an authority on religion or non-western medical therapies. I will cover what I have found to be important to patients and families in the ICU. I apologize in advance if some of the descriptions are not as nuanced as many would like. This is not meant to be a spiritual guide but an overview of spiritual issues you might encounter. If you have questions about specific issues or therapies, I encourage you to search out more comprehensive information.

Religion

Although there are many organized religions in the world, the similarities between the religions when it comes to issues around the treatment of patients far outstrip the differences. In most instances in the ICU, families go about praying and consoling each other without much interaction with the medical staff. There are a few religious beliefs that have a profound effect on the patient's health care. The most notable of these is the belief by some people who practice the faith of Jehovah's Witnesses. They have a very personal and strong belief that prohibits them from receiving any products from another human being. For this reason, they do not accept blood transfusions. Because blood transfusion is an important part of the care of many of our patients, this can have an impact on care. Although this makes my job harder as an Intensivist, I believe that their faith gives them an advantage in their healthcare that often makes up for the loss of blood transfusions as a therapeutic intervention.

Other areas of religion that can impact medical care less dramatically are dietary constraints imposed by some religious beliefs. Most hospitals have set up contingencies for dietary restrictions due to religion. Our hospital has kosher options for our Jewish community (of note, almost all tube feeding solutions and liquid meals commercially available are kosher), Halal options for our Muslim communities and fish options for those days when Catholics don't eat meat. Although these options have been well worked out for our patients, I find that the cafeterias of many hospitals are less accommodating. If you have specific dietary requirements, please tell your nurse. It is often surprising what hospital staff can do if you ask.

Although this is not connected to religion, a patient who is a firm advocate of a vegetarian diet may become physically ill at the mere thought of ingesting any meat products. Please be sure to tell the nurse and nutrition specialist about this dietary preference. In addition, vegan lifestyles often prohibit egg and egg products. Many of our medications contain egg proteins in them. It is up to the patient (or family if the patient can't make decisions) to decide how stringently to adhere to those beliefs in times of illness. It may be vitally important to know about any food allergies, such as wheat, nuts or eggs, etc., so the family should be sure the staff knows of these allergies.

The last organized religious issue that I will touch on is the issue of particular rites of passage that are performed for patients when they are sick or at the end of life. I am more familiar with the Christian rites. The most important of these is the anointing of the sick with oil (often called "last rites"). Primarily a rite of the Catholic religion, it may be as confusing to non-Catholics, as it is to members of that faith. It is the only rite, which may be performed on the same person more than once, and does ***not*** necessarily indicate that the patient is dying or will die anytime soon. Certainly, it may indicate that the patient is very ill, but many times, the patient recovers after the rites have been administered. This has been a source of confusion in the ICU on more than one occasion. A family will call a priest to see their loved one and be shocked when they find that the priest is performing last rites. The family usually comes to me to ask if I had told the priest the patient was going to die without telling the family.

In some instances, certain rites of passage, such as baptism in the Christian religions, aren't completed prior to the illness that landed the patient in the ICU in the first place. It can be a major source of comfort to a family with a seriously ill family member who has not completed all of their religion's rites of passage to have these rites performed in the hospital setting. It is no less valid in these circumstances.

Non-western methods of healing

In the last twenty years, many non-western methods of healing have become prominent. These techniques have been lumped under the names alternative therapy, complementary medicine, traditional medicine, and Eastern medicine (since many of these therapies originated in Asia). Some of these may be introduced into the Intensive Care Unit (with the permission of the health care team). In very few cases, we ask that specific therapies not be used in the ICU due to the risk of infection, or the risk of changing an important patient variable such as blood pressure. If it is not considered prudent to use a particular therapy, you are welcome to ask the specific reason. Sometimes, appropriate accommodations can be made that will allow some part

of the therapy. Some of the techniques that have been used in our ICU at the family's request are:
1) Bio feedback
2) Relaxation therapy
3) Hypnotism
4.) Reiki
5) Feng Shui
6) Acupuncture

Geography may play a large part in the popularity of some of these techniques. These are highly individualistic choices, and some physicians may be resistant to the idea of utilizing them while in the intensive care unit. If the family or the patient has had experience with any of these techniques and wishes to continue their use while in the hospital, we can only advise discussing the specifics of the therapy with the medical team. In many cases, techniques that are unfamiliar to the ICU team will be viewed with caution. In many cases, it is the patient's own positive thoughts that aid in the healing process, and anything that will encourage such positive energy is a valuable addition to the care of the patient. I make no claims for or against any of these techniques, but also recognize that some of them may be of more help to family members than to the patient.

While the hospital may be receptive to the use of any of these therapies in the ICU, the therapists will most likely not be on the hospital staff, and may be contracted through outside sources. In some cases, the hospital may be able to refer a practitioner. If this is not feasible, perhaps a website or local library may be of some assistance.

Biofeedback

Imagine if the signals by the body that are monitored by the ICU team could be used to help the patient directly. This is the premise behind biofeedback, which uses signals from inside your own body to allow you to effect certain changes. These might include: breathing patterns, altering the heart rate, decreasing anxiety, or, in its most fantastic claim, improving healing through specific techniques that can be easily taught to patients. This is how biofeedback works. Specific biofeedback therapy may require an additional monitor and even an experienced biofeedback therapist to interpret the body's signals. Not all hospitals are equipped to deal with this added therapy, but you won't know unless you ask. Some areas that may be helped by the use of biofeedback are: pain management, relaxation, and recovery from stroke in cooperation with a physical therapist. The major limitation is that the patient must be awake and able to concentrate on the task. This is not always easy for an ICU patient.

Relaxation therapy

Relaxation therapy is a close cousin to biofeedback. Instead of using internal signals to guide therapy, outside the body signals are used. Both relaxation therapy and biofeedback suffer from the limitation that the patient needs to be awake and able to follow commands to benefit from them. In the right patient, relaxation therapy can be very helpful in the treatment of anxiety. Unfortunately, a patient who is not experienced in relaxation therapy may not be able to benefit from this technique while in the intensive care unit, although it might perhaps be helpful once transferred to a less stressful location.

Relaxation therapy has been shown to decrease heart and respiration rate, to lower blood pressure, and relieve muscle tension. On occasion, it has also been known to reduce insomnia and fatigue while aiding in achieving sounder sleep.

Hypno-therapy or hypnosis

Hypno-therapy is another older method of helping patients relieve pain or stress, while allowing the body respite in order to heal itself. It has been used to good effect in recent years to help people eliminate unhealthy habits such as smoking and over-eating (and other addictive behaviors). Women have used hypnosis to reduce or alleviate labor pains. It has been shown to lessen the potential deleterious effects on the fetus by using any of the various drug-induced pain reducers. It is also useful for reducing stress, and helping the patient to manage pain on a temporary basis.

Of course, this treatment method may not work for all illnesses or patients. It may require special training on the part of the therapist in cooperation with the physician in order to achieve results. If you have questions, ask your physician for more information.

Reiki

The word Reiki may be used as a noun, an adjective or a verb, and is basically a transfer of 'life force' or energy from one being to another, or even to themselves. The practitioner is generally human, but the recipient may also be plant or animal. As in Yoga, there are degrees of understanding or training. Usually, the benefit is achieved by a direct laying on of hands, although a more advanced practitioner may be proficient in distance treatments.

There are reports of use by children for preventative medicine. Children have also been taught to teach each other. Usually, the treatment is conducted in silence, which is reputed to aid the meditative process. The entire session may take an hour or more. Reiki is considered to be spiritual in nature, but is not a religion, having originated in Japan during the early 20th Century. The laying on of hands on sick people has long been touted as a beneficial therapy in the ICU.

Feng Shui

Feng shui is an ancient Chinese philosophy that utilizes the placement of inanimate objects in the proper areas in order to achieve harmony of spirit. Doors, windows, compass points and space – all are important elements in this technique. The arrangement of furniture within a room, depending on the surrounding architectural structure is one aspect of feng shui. Adherents believe that feng shui can affect health as well as personal relationships. Some newer hospitals have become aware of this technique and implement it while constructing new intensive care units. Some may never accept it. In all cases, beds and equipment in intensive care units are placed where they are for multitudes of reasons. It is important for nothing to be changed without prior consultation with the medical staff. Inadvertently unplugging a piece of equipment can have disastrous consequences.

Acupuncture

Acupuncture is more than 2000 years old, having originated in China. This treatment involves the use of thin, metallic needles that penetrate the skin. There is scientific evidence that it is effective for use in pain management. Although it has been shown to work in many types of diseases, it is sometimes questionable for use in an intensive care unit. Because of the very nature of the ICU, where the patients are the most severely ill of any place in the hospital, the utility of acupuncture is difficult to prove. We have allowed acupuncture, and more frequently, acupressure (where pressure is applied to the points without penetrating the skin) in patients in the ICU. Many of those patients get better although it is hard to determine if acupuncture or acupressure is to credit.

Although most practitioners of acupuncture carefully sterilize their needles prior to use, the risk of infection in the ICU is so high that, for safety reasons, any device that penetrates the skin needs to be sterilized by the hospital. This limits outside practitioners from bringing needles into the ICU for acupuncture. Some hospitals, including ours, have acupuncturists employed although all the therapy in our hospital is for outpatients who come into the hospital for an appointment. Inpatient services are not yet available.

One last word on acupuncture; there are many people who claim to be acupuncture specialists with little or no training. There are formal schools and an accrediting process for acupuncture. I insist that before we even consider acupuncture for a patient, the acupuncturist must present credentials and verification of accreditation.

Making the ICU room a spiritual setting

Families are often apprehensive about putting anything in the ICU room for fear of inhibiting the ICU team's instruments. It is possible to make the room a spiritual place where the patient can get comfort and the family can find meaning. The most important first step is communicating with the nurse who is caring for your loved one. There are certain machines and/or areas in the ICU that need to be configured in a specific way. The rest of the room can perhaps be modified as long as there is room enough for everyone who needs to work in the room to be able to do so without any interference. There are a few limitations that pertain to almost all ICUs:

1) Food items pose varieties of risks for patients. Most ICUs limit food in the room, although if the patient is eating normally exceptions can be made.
2) Living plants and cut flowers carry bacteria and viruses that do not affect healthy people but may have bad consequences for patients with impaired immunity (infection fighting capacity). Most ICUs ban living plants and flowers but not artificial ones.
3) Some electronic equipment interferes with the monitoring devices in the room. Cell phones are usually banned in ICUs for this reason. Other electronic equipment may need to be checked out by the biomedical engineering department before they can be used in the ICU.
4) In addition, some ICUs restrict having anything plugged into a wall. The cords can be dangerous and most ICU rooms have a capacity for only a certain amount of electrical output and we use most of this capacity on the patient's machines. For this reason, you may be asked to bring only battery operated devices.
5) Clothing and shawls can be problematic if they interfere with the access the nurses need to the patient. Whenever possible, we try to accommodate

prayer shawls if only for during the time when the family is in the room. It is also important to tell the nurse how to handle the garment (so the nurse doesn't offend any religious sensibility).
6) Large displays are usually not possible. We have had some families that want to recreate a traditional altar in the room. This usually takes up too much space in the ICU room to be allowed. If there is a specific event that the family needs a bit more space for, this can occasionally be supported.
7) The burning of incense or candles is strictly prohibited. Medical grade oxygen that we use for our patients is potentially explosive.

There are some things I have seen patients and families do to make the room more spiritual. The most common is to hang pictures of loved ones or of religious icons. This is a common enough request that most ICU rooms have a corkboard or a window where there is room. Music in the room is another way to improve the environment. Often softly playing music is not a problem in the ICU. Some families bring in headphones for patients to use. This is usually OK but should be cleared by the nurse. Prayer shawls and pins of religious or spiritual significance are often 'placed' on patients, but not attached to them or their garments.

The most effective way of making the room more spiritual in my opinion is having people in the room who can pray, chant or meditate with the patient. Some families will have different people from the community come in and pray with the patient every hour or so. This can change the environment in the room greatly. Just be sure to check with the nurse before starting and make sure to honor visiting hours if your hospital has them.

Resources

Almost all hospitals have some protocols in place to comfort patients in a spiritual way. In our hospital, we have a chaplaincy service. The chaplains are available for all patients and coordinate all of our other spiritual programs. There are specific programs in our hospital for the more common religious beliefs (specifically, Christianity, Judaism, and Islam) such as prayer services or areas for daily prayer. If you come from a less common tradition, it may be harder to find specific programs. Talk to the chaplain and see if any arrangements can be made.

If the patient is hospitalized close to home, then he may derive additional comfort from a visit by his own clergyperson. Such visits are easily arranged by the family or the hospital chaplaincy service. If hospitalized away from home, a representative of the patient's own faith may be readily available, as well. Especially in larger hospitals, Chaplains are available 24/7. (This may not be the case in some smaller hospitals.) These chaplains are trained in all religions, not just their own, but they also have a current list of chaplains from other faiths. They can call on these chaplains from other faiths if requested.

Non-traditional families
Times have changed, as has the very definition of the word 'family.' It is not uncommon for a couple to be deeply committed to each other without the formality of marriage vows. Adoption between races is becoming more usual with every passing day. So, too, are couples that are not the traditional heterosexual pairing.

Not all families will experience any of these (or other) groupings. I urge caution and temperance while in the ICU, for any relationships that may seem *different* to you. If your family does contain a non-traditional pairing, the ICU is not the place for avoidance or preventing visitation that may well be beneficial to the patient. This is especially true if the patient is in such a relationship. To be deprived of the comfort of a loving partner while fighting for one's life, is to have added yet more insurmountable objects along the pathway toward good health.

There are multiple reasons why the patient might not be able to speak while in the ICU, however, once the patient has recovered and is no longer in the hospital setting, he can make his own opinions known. It is fairly easy to arrange visitation so as to not have contentious visitors appear at the same time. In the long run, everyone will benefit from letting cooler heads prevail. The object is, after all, the well-being and return to good health of the patient.

Chapter Six

<u>The Browns</u>

Nurse Mark and the Intensivist were conferring with Alex and Tom. Mark had the ever-present clipboard in his hands. The doctor spoke. "I want you to know, Mr. Brown, we're doing everything we know of to do for your wife. We want to be hopeful, but it may be a few more hours yet before we'll really be certain. We'll continue treating her aggressively for as long as we need to."

"We need to be prepared, however, and these are tough questions," Mark said. "I know they're hard, but for her sake, they need to be asked." He looked at both Alex and Tom, then nodded his head once more. He looked at the top sheet on the clipboard. "Has she ever expressed any opinions about extreme treatment? What should be done in a situation like the one we're in now? What would she want us to do? We want to do what she would want, as much as we can. But what is good for one patient might be totally wrong for another."

"Oh. Can you be more explicit?" asked Tom.

"We don't know what's happening just yet. It may be a heart attack or a brain attack – "

Tom looked at Alex and said, "Stroke. He means she might be paralyzed." Alex buried his head in his hands. "And if so, then what happens?" continued Tom.

"She might spend years in that condition."

Tom sat up straighter. "A nursing home? Is that what you're talking about? Not my Mom. No way."

Alex gawked at his step-son. "But she'd still be alive, right?"

"Alex. I go into nursing homes all the time. Mom wouldn't want to be there, believe me, and you wouldn't want her there, either."

"But she'd still be alive, right?"

"*You* might call it that. *I* wouldn't. And I don't

think she would, either."

"Has Mrs. Brown ever talked about quality of life issues with either of you?" Mark asked. "Each person generally has some idea of what they want for themselves, which may not be what another person would choose. You can't choose her opinions for her. That's why I asked about an Advanced Directive."

"I doubt if she's ever thought of it. She's too young to think of such things," Alex responded.

"No, Mr. Brown. Age has nothing to do with it. Illness is no respecter of age. I mean no disrespect to you or her or anyone in the family, but we may need to make some hard decisions here, and it's best to be at least somewhat prepared. I'll leave you for a while, so you may discuss as you will, in private."

Speaking for the Patient

A very important point for families to remember is that all the health care workers in the hospital, the doctors, nurses, therapists, even the housekeepers work for the patient. Although the healthcare providers make decisions about appropriate treatments and implement them, they are supposed to make those decisions based on what the patient wants us to do. More plainly, in America, you have a say in what happens to your body. If you are presented with a medical problem, such as a cancer, that requires surgery to correct, you have the right to refuse that surgery. As doctors, we may believe strongly that the surgery is the right thing to do, but we must still respect the wishes of the patient. The same thing occurs in the intensive care unit. If a patient refuses a type of therapy, it is incumbent on the doctor to abide by the wishes of the ICU patient.

People are admitted to the ICU because they are gravely ill. Even if the prognosis for recovery in the ICU is good, patients are at high risk for complications, which can lead to a poor outcome. For this reason, it is important for patients and families to consider what to do if your loved one has to face the prospect of death. This takes on an added sense of urgency if the patient is unable to speak for him (or her) self, either because they have a breathing tube in place or cannot talk or if they are unconscious. In that situation, the family (or the person designated by the patient to speak for them) now becomes the agent for the patient to make sure that his/her wishes are kept.

In the ICU, trying to have the patient or the family decide about every single therapy becomes very difficult. There are so many things going on at once that it would be impossible to give good care if we had to stop and ask the patient – or family – about every single intervention. There are times when a delay for this purpose can prove fatal. Instead, we like to get an idea of the patient's goals and make decisions appropriately.

For example, if a patient who has chronic breathing problems from emphysema comes into the ICU, we may have a discussion based on what types of outcomes are appropriate. The patient may say "Do whatever you can to make me better, but if I deteriorate to the point where I need a breathing machine, I would rather die in comfort than live my life on a ventilator."

This would then define the limits of the care we can provide and allow us as doctors and nurses to make a whole bunch of decisions to help the patient get better without having to ask permission for every medication and procedure up to the limit of having the breathing tube placed. This is what I like to call "Synchronizing the Goals". When the patient's goals and the care team goals are synchronized, the patient can get the best care possible without receiving care that is too aggressive or that might leave the patient with a quality of life he might find not acceptable.

I think that a very important issue to discuss right up front is **quality of life**. This term is often thrown around casually on television and in hospitals without any real understanding of what it means. Modern medicine is better than ever at keeping patients alive. We have machines to make you breathe, medicines to keep your blood pressure up or drop it down, and special beds that rotate to make sure a patient doesn't develop bedsores. Fortunately, today, the 'end of life' supposition often ends up *not* being the end of that person's life. Although this is great news on the whole, it is a bit problematic for some patients who are faced with profound disabilities after we "save their life". In the 1920's and 30's, this problem was seen most frequently with polio patients. They would most likely be left neurologically disabled if we were able to keep them alive. This was a slightly different scenario than the current type of patient we see in the ICU: one who is substantially older and with more medical problems than the victims of the polio epidemic.

This leads to the question of whether to continue aggressive care for a patient who has lived a long life and is facing a long debilitating illness if they survive. In America (Canada, the United States and Mexico), a great deal of weight is placed on the patient's wishes: Is the patient's preference for **quality** of life or **quantity** of life? This can be a very difficult situation for a family member who is trying to make decisions for a loved one in the ICU who can't speak for themselves.

As a good example of how this quality of life vs. quantity of life issue can color decisions, I (JP) often use my own family. My mother is very active despite being in her 80s. She continues to chase after grandchildren, cook for every group that asks her to, and visit friends who are less fortunate than she is. She has told me that if she can't cook breakfast for my family and me in the morning when we come to visit, what good would life be? My father, despite the fact that he has been married to my mother for almost 50 years and lives in the same house, has told me that as long as he can feel the warmth of the sun on his face, he wants to be alive. So you can see, if I was making decisions for my mother and my father, I would likely have to choose different options for each of them based on their wishes.

Some people with foresight or because of previous medical problems have thought about this situation and have made their wishes known. There are four ways that a family member or a physician will know if the patient has thought about those issues: 1) They have spoken to family members about their wishes, 2) they have filled out an advanced directive at the time of their hospital admission describing what they want, 3) they have filled out a Living will, or 4) they have designated someone to be their durable power of attorney for healthcare. We will discuss each of these in turn. After, we will discuss what to do if your family member hasn't done any of these things (which is most commonly the case).

1) The patient has talked about what to do if there is a life-threatening situation.

Many people have had casual conversations usually around news stories that go something like this: "Don't leave me as a vegetable. If I ever get that bad, pull the plug." Unfortunately, the devil is in the details. Does being a vegetable mean having a stroke that leaves you paralyzed on one side of your body but allows you to talk and interact with your family? Does it mean not being able to talk and understand what people around you are saying? Does it mean not being able to care for yourself, leaving you in a nursing home? Most people only think in general terms because they cannot imagine a future with a horrible illness. In actuality, when push comes to shove and you are presented with a life-threatening illness, many people think differently about their circumstances. I find that people often look at situations and say "I wouldn't want to live like that" where I think the more important phrasing is "If I was in that situation, I would rather die than have any heroic effort expended to keep me alive."

Often, families find that either no one has had an explicit conversation with the patient about their wishes or that many people in the family have had some variation of the conversation. Almost no families have discussed the specific situation in which they find themselves. As such, families are often left to put together the conversations and the life experiences of the patient to come up with a determination of what they would want done.

A good example of this comes to mind from my training. A patient who had severe emphysema developed pneumonia and was admitted to the ICU with breathing difficulty. The infection spread to the rest of his body causing a blood clot in his leg. Prior to his hospitalization, he was very debilitated – unable to leave his house for any amount of time (only to get to his doctor's appointments). He was heavily sedated to make his breathing easier. The family was faced with the decision of whether to amputate his leg, which would have likely saved his life or to make him comfortable so that he didn't suffer discomfort or indignity at the end of his life. He had spoken to his wife and his brother about not wanting to be in a nursing home but also said he was afraid of dying. Lately, he had made statements about how tiring it was to not know if his next breath was coming.

The physicians, nurses and family had a family meeting to decide what the right course of action was for him. After presenting all the medical facts, the question I raised was "What do you think he would want us to do?" The family put their heads together and discussed all of the times he had talked about what kind of care he would like. They found that none of the discussed situations really looked like his current situation. They decided that given his conversations and the way he lived his life, he would find his current situation unacceptable. This was the information they needed to make decisions about how to move forward.

2) The patient has filled out an advanced directive.
Many hospitals have advanced directive forms that they offer to all patients. These forms don't necessarily follow a standard format but they all have the same goal. They discuss types of medications that patients do and don't want to have. For example, many advanced directive forms have a section asking whether the patient would want to have a blood transfusion if the doctor feels it is necessary. There are also places on most forms to discuss whether the patient would like to have a breathing machine or other therapies should they become necessary.

The advantage of the advanced directive is that the patient fills it out when they are coming into the hospital for a specific problem or procedure. If you are coming into the hospital for artery surgery in your neck, it is easier to say "I would not like to have a breathing machine if I have a large stroke after my procedure." This would have greatly eased the task of my patient's family mentioned above. Instead of having to determine the wishes of their loved one from other conversations, the family would have had more direct information.

The major disadvantage to advanced directives in the hospital is that many patients who come to the ICU are in no condition to fill out the forms when they come into the hospital. In addition, many patients who come in to the hospital for elective surgery choose to think the best and forget the worst.

Don't automatically overlook an older document that has been signed by the patient. Unless there is a more current version of the same instructions, this older copy can still serve a useful purpose, by exposing the patient's thoughts on a given topic.

3) The patient has filled out a Living Will

Living wills are written versions of the first situation. They substitute for a good conversation with family about what you want and don't want done if you become terminally ill. The major drawback to a living will is that the language sounds as though it was written by a contract lawyer (not a physician or a patient). Every state has a living will document that is standard. (You can reference http://liv-will1.uslivin.com/forms.html for your state's form.)

Most of them include terminology that sounds like this: "If two doctors independently determine that I am unconscious from an irreversible and terminal cause and that there is no chance that I will ever regain consciousness, I don't want. . ."

This is fine for those patients who are diagnosed with cancer. They are much less helpful if, for instance, you are dying of emphysema. In that instance, you clearly have a life-threatening illness and you may not be able to survive without a breathing machine, but you do not qualify for directives made under your living will. There is nothing to say that you may not come out of your coma for a period of time before you die. I usually tell families that living wills are important if your loved one is diagnosed with cancer – *specifically*. This kind of document is also important because it means that the patient has thought about their life and decided what types of therapy they want. This usually leads to the types of discussions that are very helpful in the first scenario "**The patient has talked about what to do if there is a life-threatening situation**".

4) The patient has designated someone to be their durable power of attorney for healthcare.

Some people will designate a person whom they trust as their durable power of attorney. This is a fully formed legal document that must be signed in the presence of a lawyer or a notary, in order to be legal. Basically, the patient, in advance of becoming a patient, designates someone they know and trust as a spokesperson for them if they are in a condition where they cannot speak for themselves. This person can be a family member or work colleague. Because this is a legal arrangement, it is enforceable. If the person who is setting up the power of attorney is smart, they will have a long discussion about what is appropriate and what is not appropriate care.

The one potential drawback of this type of arrangement is that it supersedes all other legal arrangements including marriage. So if you designate your best friend as the durable power of attorney when you cannot speak for yourself, then that person, not your wife or husband, will make decisions on your behalf to the healthcare team.

Accessing the forms.

Filling out forms and setting up legal arrangements is meaningful only when the documents of these transactions are available. I cannot tell you how many times we talk to family members and decide care issues only to have them later present us with a living will or durable power of attorney they just found in a drawer in the house.

Care decision forms should ideally be done while a person is in good health, and can make sensible decisions. Be sure family members know where these papers are located (If they can't be found, they're not very helpful.) Conversely, if you have a family member in the ICU who you think has a care decision form, you should send someone to look for it. Social workers in most hospitals can help you by describing the forms, finding lawyers who may have submitted the forms or filling out new forms.

A living will is also subject to the laws of the state in which the patient resides. If you move to another state after having completed such a document, be certain it is still valid in your new state. Your family doctor should have a copy, as well as your spouse or responsible family member, and possibly your attorney. Locked away in a safety deposit box is not necessarily a good place for the only copy to be! (Check with an attorney or Bar Association in your state of residence for complete particulars, although you may not need an attorney to execute the document. In some states, a notary public or two unrelated adult persons may witness your signature. To reference your state laws, please visit this helpful website for assistance: http://www.uslwr.com/default.asp)

In the end, all of these mechanisms are in place to help patients and families get the care that they really want. The best way for this to occur is to communicate well between family members. If your family member is in the ICU and is still able to talk intelligently – and intelligibly – it is worthwhile to have a discussion about what their specific wishes are if things were to get worse. Again, Social workers in the hospital can help decide what form of directive is best and what forms need to be filled out.

Other End of Life issues

Futility
There are times that even with our advanced medical technology; we are unable to save a person's life. Or, in some cases we are able to save the patient's life but not in a way that allows the patient to have a type of life they are willing to accept. When the goals that the patient is trying to meet (whether it is living or living independently) are out of reach of our technology, we consider the care to be futile.

Doctors and nurses have a good idea of when the care we offer is no longer heading to an acceptable outcome for the patient. Patients' families often do not have the medical knowledge to understand. I find this can be one of the most difficult interactions between a physician and a patient or family member.

A good example of this comes from a patient I took care of recently. The patient came into the hospital with heart failure. It was determined that he would need a heart transplant to survive. He was put on a type of artificial heart until he could be transplanted. Before he could get his transplant, however, he had a cardiac arrest that caused severe brain damage. This brain damage was so severe that he would not be able to tolerate the medicines that he would have to take for the heart transplant. He had specific wishes that he not be kept on permanent life support. His problem was tragic; he would never get well enough to qualify for a new heart. He clearly didn't want to be hooked up to life support for the rest of his life. The care we were giving was clearly futile. The obvious choice was to stop the artificial heart and let him pass away peacefully. It took his family weeks to come to the same realization that the physicians and nurses made in the first 4 days.

How a doctor or nurse approaches the family about futile care is very important. Some families feel as though they are asked to "pull the plug". I can't speak for anyone else, but I really dislike the term "pull the plug". First there is no plug to pull, second, it suggests that we stop caring for patients when we change our goal to comfort which is far from the truth, and third, I personally wouldn't care if my mother had to go to a nursing home, I would be happy to simply have her alive in whatever condition she would be in. Therefore, if it were up to me, I would never let the doctors remove care. But that would not be my mother's wish.

The way I approach families is to ask them "If I could ask your loved one – if they were awake and I could ask them – would they want to continue if they were in this situation, what would they say? Whatever you tell me, I will use as a basis on which to form my decision, but I will not be asked to 'pull the plug'. Your part is to tell me what they would want me to do." Families often find it much easier to describe what their loved one would and wouldn't want if the responsibility weren't weighted with the thought of 'pulling the plug'. As doctors, we are entrusted to do as much as we can for patients, but we don't expect them to understand absolutely everything. We ask families to give us the sense of what the patient wants and then it's up to the physician with his or her expertise to say how we will meet the goals the patient has set up through his or her family.

Do not resuscitate orders and comfort care

Some patient have made it clear by one of the mechanisms above or the family has decided that based on how the patient lived their life, aggressive care will not achieve an acceptable goal for the patient. In these patients, we write an order called **DNR (do not resuscitate)**. This alerts all doctors and nurses that if something catastrophic happens like the patient's heart stops beating, aggressive therapies such as shocking the patient, putting in a breathing tube or surgery are not warranted.

This order is important because when someone's heart stops in the ICU, the nearest doctors and nurses will respond. These people may never have met your loved one and don't have an understanding of what the patient's wishes are. Having a form on the chart that alerts these doctors and nurses that the person doesn't want heroic measures prevents unnecessary and undignified procedures being done on a patient who wouldn't want those things done. A DNR can be requested by the patient at any time to any doctor during the hospitalization.

Comfort care is a bit different. Sometimes when a patient is so severely disabled that they will never make an adequate recovery, the family chooses to make the patient comfortable either with medicines, extended family visitation or physical comfort measures. This allows a family to spend the last hours of their loved one's life with them in privacy. There are a host of therapies (including removal of the breathing machine and blood pressure medicines) that can make a patient more comfortable if they are at the end of their natural life. In addition, there are palliative care physicians at most hospitals who specialize in caring for the needs of terminally ill patients. They can be a valuable help in determining a treatment plan to keep the patient comfortable.

Death by Neurological Criteria (a.k.a. Brain Death)

One of the most complicated things to understand in the ICU is when your doctor comes and tells you that your loved one is "brain dead". In the outside world, we use the term brain dead to mean that we are thoughtless or not intelligent. Many patients' families have misconceptions about what brain death means.

The clearest explanation of brain death is the term "Death by Neurological Criteria" (the term favored by many doctors now.) In the days before intensive care units, we diagnosed death when someone's heart and lungs stopped. So if a person had a catastrophic brain injury and his or her brain stopped working, his or her heart and lungs would also stop working and the diagnosis would be clear. Once we started using breathing machines (ventilators) and medicines to keep hearts beating, the progression from the brain dying to heart and lungs stopping was interrupted. For this reason, the medical community decided that we needed to develop a way to diagnose the patient whose brain was dead, but that we as doctors were keeping the body moving mechanically. A panel of distinguished doctors and ethicists at Harvard's medical school put together a list of tests and criteria by which we could be certain that a patient was actually dead even though his heart and lungs were still working. So you see, the diagnosis of death is now made differently than previously (by heart and lungs not working) by neurological criteria.

Over the last fifty years, death by neurological criteria has become accepted in almost every country in the world. In all states in the United States, death by neurological criteria is accepted as legal death (Two states, New Jersey and New York allow families who for religious reasons object to the diagnosis of death by neurological criteria to wait for the heart and lungs to stop before declaring the patient dead). This has become a way to determine when patients have reached a point where their brain is irreversibly broken so that families can begin grieving without holding out false hope that their loved one will recover.

Chapter 7

Organ Donation

The Browns avoid a difficult decision

The normally-ebullient Marcia (Olivia's sister) had been quiet and morose since Olivia's condition had become so unstable. Both her husband Blair, and her nephew Tom approached her, offering consolation for whatever difficulty she was experiencing. Stubbornly, she remained silent, until at last, she wailed, "It was Mary! Such a horrible decision she had to make. What if that had happened to us, too?"

The room became suddenly quiet. None of the others had any notion of what she meant – or even about whom she was speaking.

Blair asked, "What *are* you talking about? Who is Mary?"

Between tears, Marcia made a valiant attempt to control her voice. "Mary is my new friend – we met in the waiting room last week. It was her husband who died two days ago. She had to decide what to do about organ donation." A shudder shook her body as she shredded the tissue in her hand. "I don't know why they had to bother her about such things at such a time."

Tom came over to kneel down in front of her. Taking one of her hands in his, he clasped it tightly, and spoke gently to her. "Aunt Marcia. Please listen to me. Haven't you ever seen those bumper stickers that say, "Donate your organs. Heaven knows you won't need them again." The seeming *non sequitur* surprised the other inhabitants in the room.

"What are you talking about!" someone said.

"It's a very important consideration for a person to make. Any organs that aren't affected by the illness or cause of death can extend the life of a recipient, if the harvesting is done properly. Haven't you all been asked about organ donation when you renewed your driver's license last time around?"

He continued. "Generally, this decision is made by an individual before they become ill or are in an accident. It doesn't always work out that way, but thousands of lives are saved every year by organ donation. I've signed up for it, and Mom and I have discussed it, but I don't know if she ever followed through on it." He turned to look at his step-father. "Do you know, Alex?"

Alex did not want to even think of such a thing at a time like this, and he turned away from the family, disgust showing on his face.

"It's entirely voluntary, you know." Tom patted Marcia's hand and stood up.

"That's what I was trying to say, but the words wouldn't come out right," Marcia stammered. "Mary told me that her husband wanted to be a donor, but he'd not managed to sign the papers as yet, so she had to make the decision for him the other night. It bothered her a lot, until Father Malone was able to comfort her and then a really sympathetic young woman from the organ donation place explained what they could and couldn't do. It all seemed so easy and so . . . so, um – useful?" She paused long enough to have a swallow of the water Tom held out to her.

"This woman told her that a dozen – or more – other people could be helped by the donation of several of his organs. They even knew several people who had been on a donor list, but some of them had died while still waiting." Marcia smiled briefly. "Mary said it suddenly seemed very much like the right thing to do. So she signed the papers." Marcia reached for Blair's hand. "I think I'm going to do this, too," she stated. "I hope you don't mind," she said, looking up at him. "I love you enough to want to make it easier for you when that time comes. But that doesn't mean that you have, to, too – unless you want to, of course."

"Oh! I can't do this!" wailed Alex, as he began to pace, furiously, around the small room. "I don't know what to do. What to say. We've never discussed these things. Not ever."

"Mr. Brown?" A young woman, unfamiliar to Alex and Tom interrupted the conversation. Dr. Charles was one of the young resident doctors, working towards becoming an Intensivist. She repeated, "I thought you'd want to know. Mrs. Brown is responding again. She seems to have turned the corner. She's stabilized."

"Oh, thank God," Alex cried, tears running boldly down his face. The other men in the room came to console him, their tears mingling with his.

Making something good from the worst day of your life

When a person dies, it is usually a very sad experience. Depending on the type of illness (chronic or sudden) and your beliefs about the afterworld, there may be some comfort in the thought that your loved one is no longer suffering or in a better place. Regardless of your feelings, organ donation can add a little more meaning to the loss of a loved one. The best example we have of this comes from me (Kelly). This letter was in response to a newspaper columnist who had written about the life-and-death decisions made during March, 2005, regarding Terry Schiavo, who had severe brain-damage, and had been on a feeding tube for more than a decade.

"My darling daughter died on October 29, (2004) having not been ill or anything other than healthy, to the best of our collective knowledge. 'Our' being her husband, her brother and me. She was 12 days short of her 45th birthday.

It seems as though the sun has gone out of my life, but every now and then it does briefly peek out to brighten a moment or two. Because I am a writer, I wrote a tribute to her, which I sent out to friends and family located around the world. Several of her friends asked for a copy, which I happily provided. In this tribute, I mentioned that even though Kristi is now gone from us, she still lives, because, although she had not executed a will, she had told both her husband and me that she wanted to be an organ donor.

Unfortunately, because of the time spent by the EMT crew in trying to resuscitate her at home, and then at the hospital, very little of the more usual harvesting could be done. However, the doctors were able to take her femurs, hip joints, some heart valves and pieces of arteries. It sounds grotesque to list these dearly loved parts of her in this way, but until this time, I had no idea they could even be considered for such donations.

She also had lovely long brown hair, very curly, never permed or colored. The day after the viewing, before the cremation, her hair was braided and cut, to be given to "Locks of Love". This donation came about, in part, because she and her husband were members of a motorcycle club, of which the members regularly donate their long hair to this organization. It is similar in nature to "Wigs for Kids" in providing wigs for children and teens who have lost their own hair due to chemotherapy or other medical intervention. Kristi was the impetus behind several such donations in recent years, so it seemed only fitting that she should also join those ranks.

I miss her terribly, and nothing can take her place in my heart. But yet, it does provide some ease to know that because of her unselfishness, a few other fortunate folks out there will benefit from her gift to them.

Please keep reminding your readers that the gift of life and love can last a long time, even if only in a mother's heart."

Organ Donation

When a patient dies either by their heart stopping or by declaration of death by neurological criteria, organ donation of some kind is usually possible. For patients who die from a disease that causes their heart to stop, there is the option of donating hair, bone, and parts of the eye (cornea). In addition, some patients have wishes that their bodies be used in the education of training doctors. This type of donation is called whole body donation. In our institution, the medical school accepts whole body donation for the training of medical students and post-graduate residents. At the end of the school year, there is a very nice memorial ceremony for all the people who have donated their bodies for education. Some institutions have a "Wall of Honor" on which are small plaques bearing the name of each individual donor. *(From Kelly: My daughter's paternal grandparents are memorialized in this way at the University of Michigan.)*

Donation after Declaration of Death by Neurological Criteria (DNC) or Brain Death

For patients who meet the criteria for death because of neurological injury, organ donation can be a bigger gift. In addition to donating bone, hair and eyes, patients can decide to donate solid organs as well. Liver, kidneys, heart, pancreas, small intestines and lungs can be donated to patients who need them to survive.

The process for organ donation in patients who are dead by neurological criteria can be confusing. First, the physician comes and talks to the family about the diagnosis and what it means (that the person is legally, morally and actually dead). After the family has had all of their questions answered, a doctor with a representative of an organ procurement organization (OPO) will come to the family and explain the option of organ donation. If the patient has previously expressed the wish to be a donor or the family feels this is what the patient would choose, paper work is filled out to consent to the procedure. The patient is then sent to the operating room and the organs are procured and sent to places where patients are in need of them.

Donation after Declaration of Death by Cardiac Arrest (DCD)

There is another type of organ donation that has recently become more common. This type of donation called "Donation after Cardiac Death" also allows the patient to donate solid organs like the liver and kidneys. In this type of donation, after a family has decided to change the focus of care to comfort care, an organ donation specialist approaches the family about organ donation. If the family (or patient) consents and the patient meets certain criteria, they are taken to the operating room where the life-sustaining interventions are stopped. When the person is declared dead by conventional means (no heart or lung activity), the doctors quickly recover the organs and send them to patients who will benefit.

How do you know if someone wanted to be an organ donor?

Just like the decision about care at the end of life, this is a very personal decision. In all states in the United States, the bureau of motor vehicles asks drivers to decide whether they would want to be organ donors should the situation occur. This registration is a very helpful indicator of the patient's wishes. In many states (including Ohio where we live), if a person signs up as an organ donor through their driver's license, the hospital uses this information as a binding declaration of the patient's intent to donate their organs.

To say this in plain English, if you go to the bureau of motor vehicles, sign up as an organ donor and subsequently get into a car accident that leaves you dead by neurological criteria (brain dead), your drivers license is your permission to donate your organs. This has the advantage of not putting the family in the situation of having to decide whether donation is what the patient wants.

If there are no predetermined wishes on which to base our decision, it is the responsibility of the family to decide if organ donation is what the patient would want. I had a sad story that illustrates this point very well. A 65-year-old woman came into my ICU with a massive bleed in her brain. She quickly progressed to brain death. Her durable power of attorney was a long-standing gentleman friend who was at her bedside during her entire hospital stay. When we discussed brain death with him, he told us he was familiar with the topic and had no questions.

When the representative from our organ procurement agency, LifeBanc, came to discuss the donation, she recognized the gentleman immediately. It turns out, a month before; his only son (an adult) had died in another hospital after a car accident. This man had agreed to have his son be an organ donor based on the reasoning that his son was a veteran of the Gulf war and always devoted himself to selfless acts like joining the military. When the question came to deciding whether his lady friend would want to donate, he politely declined saying "she never really gave to charity and she wasn't interested in helping people other than her direct family." In effect, the same person faced with the same decision made two different choices based on what he thought the patient would want. This is a good example of an excellent advocate for a family member.

Ultimately, the ability to improve or save someone else's life when yours is unsalvageable is a very noble goal. Like I said in the letter above, it often gives the family some peace to know that as tragic an incident as the loss of a loved one can still do some good to someone. There are thousands of patients in the world waiting for transplantable organs. We need more organs to be able to save as many people as we can. This obviously is a secondary concern when a patient still has a chance to survive; but when all hope of recovery is lost, helping others is a good thing.

What is the process for donation?

Each hospital has a different way of approaching a family about donation. This is how we do it, which I think is pretty typical for hospitals around the country. Typically, when a patient is declared dead by neurological criteria, the medical team sits down with the family to discuss the passing of their loved one. As you might expect (except for anyone having read this book), the concept of "brain death" is difficult to explain to a grieving family.

After the ICU team has discussed the situation with the family and all their questions are answered, a specialist from the organ procurement organization (OPO) sit down with the family and discuss whether donation is in the patient's wishes. Usually, the specialist already knows if the patient has signed up as an organ donor through their driver's license. If the patient has decided through the driver's license or the family believes that donation is what the patient would want, then the process of donation begins. (To reference your state's laws, please visit this helpful website for assistance: http://www.uslwr.com/default.asp)

Before donation can occur, a number of tests need to be done to make sure that the patient's organs are suitable for donation and the patient doesn't harbor any diseases that could harm the person who would receive the organ. This process can take up to a day to complete. Usually, we are able to get all the information we need within about 12 hours. At that time, the patient is taken to the operating room where the organs are recovered and sent to patients who need them.

The family generally gets a thank you note from the organ procurement organization that explains what happened to the organs. Names of the recipients are seldom included in the information in order to protect their privacy. In some cases, families have asked to meet the recipients of their loved one's organs. This can sometimes be arranged through the OPO if both the family and the recipients are in agreement. Other types of communication may occur if both parties are in agreement; the OPO is almost always the preferred conduit.

On a personal note, I have seen patients and families whose lives have been amazingly improved (and in some cases, prolonged) by organ donation. The effect that a kidney transplant can have on a person who otherwise would be damned to dialysis three times a week, or the liver transplant patient who would die without a transplant is incalculable. We need more organs for transplantation to meet the need of the patients for whom new organs could mean a return to a more normal life. When it is your family member who is dead, it is sometimes difficult to feel good about someone else getting a benefit when you are suffering. Later, I suspect that some families regret that their gut response was to not donate organs.

Chapter Eight

The Browns

Carolyn at 13 considers herself to be all grown-up. Except she's not grown-up enough to want to continue playing 'Mom' to her two younger brothers. 'When is Mom coming home?' is the main topic of her conversation. She's curious about the hospital and the ICU (having heard so much talk about the place) and if truth be known, she misses her Mom. A lot. She's no longer a child – why can't she go see her Mom? What's the hang-up, here, anyway?

Alex, Jr. at 11 is on the cusp of continually undecided. He is very athletic and when presented with any kind of ball he knows instinctively what to do with or about it. He certainly loves his Mom a great deal, but isn't too sure about seeing her confined to a bed. He's seen a couple of 'hospital shows' on TV, and they're scary! But still, he's almost a man! Shouldn't he be able to handle all this? Will Carolyn get on his case if he doesn't go? Lucky Ben. He's too young to go!

Ben at 6 is young for his age, and he knows absolutely that he does not want to go to the hospital for any reason whatever. Not even to see his dearly-loved Mom in the ICU. He's heard talk about when she's moved to a more normal place in the hospital, and thinks maybe that might be better. But he's still not sure. He's never seen his Mom in bed like this before, and he's not sure he wants to now, either! As the 'baby' of the family, he may well feel closer to his Mom than the other children, having her to himself more often in his first five years.

All three of the Brown children are in good health – Olivia has seen to that through the years. Carolyn, as the oldest child, has a maturity that belies her years. Alex, Jr., is pretty much normal boy of his age. Both children are intelligent and curious about the world around them, in addition to being well behaved and obedient. There is little doubt that they could visit their Mom with no serious repercussions.

It is only Ben who causes feelings of concern in this regard. As curious and intelligent as the older children are, he is not as mature at the age of six as either of them was. At times, he cries easily, and is not at all sure he really wants to go to the hospital for any reason whatever. Gentle questioning by Father Malone reveals that all the emphasis on behaving well at the hospital has caused Ben great concern. ("If you're *very good*, you can go see your Mother.") Finally, in tears, he asks, "What if I can't be good enough? Will that make Mama worse?"

Father Malone has the wisdom to understand the little boy's fears, and reassure him on several levels. Since the doctors have told the family that Olivia is expected to be transferred to a regular medical unit in another week or so, the priest suggests that Ben's visit wait until that happens. Seeing his Mom in a less restrictive setting will make life much easier for all concerned.

Ben visibly relaxes after the priest's visit, becoming the happy, cheerful little boy he's always been. Even though he and Olivia miss each other dreadfully, a visit in a less tense surrounding will be much better for everyone, and have a happier outcome.

Children in the ICU

It is very difficult to know whether to allow children to visit their adult loved ones in the ICU. Frequently, parents come to me and the nurses or other staff in the ICU with questions about whether to allow children in to see their loved ones. This can be especially crucial if the patient is a parent and there is a concern for the patient's life. On one hand, the family often feels the child may miss the opportunity to see their parent for the last time. On the other hand, they worry about traumatizing the child with the sight of a sick parent in the ICU.

In my experience there are four issues that go into the question of whether a child should be allowed to visit patients in the ICU: 1) How will the visit affect the child, 2) How will the visit from the child affect the patient, 3) Will having children in the ICU be disruptive to other patients or healthcare workers, and 4) are there realistic risks of children contracting infections in the ICU setting?

How will the visit affect the child?

At what age are children old enough to be exposed to the potentially scarring environment of the ICU? I have asked this question of child psychiatrists. Each of them replied that as all children are different in their maturity and previous experience, there is no set guideline. However, I find that before the age of seven, most children have a hard time understanding the concept of a gravely ill family member in all its complexity.

As children get older, they are more aware of the concepts of illness and the possibility of losing their loved ones. At some point, the balance tips from lack of understanding to understanding. Younger children may be traumatized by the sight of their loved one in the ICU, but will not understand what is happening if they don't get to visit. At an older age, the trauma of the ICU is more manageable but the children may fantasize the worst scenario if they don't get to see for themselves. Although that transition seems to happen around seven years of age with most children, some make the transition earlier rather than later. Generally speaking, a parent is the best judge of a child's maturity level, and thus is best able to make the determination if that child should be permitted to visit a patient in the ICU.

One of the most important ways to determine if your child is really aware of what is going on in the ICU is to sit down and talk. Ask the child in an open-ended way why their loved one is in the hospital. If they know, ask what they think is going to happen. Ask them how they feel about going to the hospital. If they say they are scared or seem apprehensive, you should be very careful about how you proceed. Professional help can be very valuable in situations where the child doesn't understand or is apprehensive.

In pediatric care (children with diseases) there has been a great deal of study into how brothers and sisters cope with visitation. The research shows that both siblings and patients do better if they are allowed to visit even at young ages. This may not apply to the child visiting an adult (especially a parent) because the parent is an authority figure and thoughts of death may not only engender feelings of loss but also worry about stability of the home environment and of support. This is to say, if a brother is sick and in the hospital, the thought of him dying will make a child sad. But, if it is a father, it also comes with the fear of being sent to live with relatives or in foster care, loss of family money, and worries about the future stability of the family.

If you have questions about your child's ability to cope with the visit, I recommend that that you first talk to the social workers in the hospital to find a child psychologist to help your loved one. Although there are other resources like child welfare specialists that are sometimes available to work with children visiting the hospital, they seldom have the resources to follow the children for an extended period of time after the hospital stay. Child welfare specialists may be appropriate but they should be under the guidance of a psychologist.

If there has been a death or funeral of a loved one or neighbor within the previous six months, it might be even more important to discuss in advance. This sort of recent memory is only too likely to become transposed in the child's mind, leaving them vulnerable to additional fears. A child that is highly emotional or easily brought to excessive tears might actually be harmed by visiting at such a time.

How will the visit from the child affect the patient?

I have been unable to find any research to suggest that patients get a benefit from *or* are harmed by children visiting them in the hospital. Perhaps this is because the reasoning behind such visits is very complicated. Is it the patient who most wants the visit? Or another member of the family? Or even the child? I have spoken to a number of patients in the ICU about whether they want their children to visit. About half of the people I talk to would like to have them visit and the other half would not. The most common responses include "I wouldn't want them to see me like this," "My children give me strength; just seeing them will help me improve," "I wouldn't want to burden my children with my illness," "I don't want my children's scared faces to be my memory of them in the ICU; I would rather remember them happy and at home," "I would like to have my children visit so that I can show them that I am alright. (Or going to be alright.)"

People have very strong opinions about how they raise their children and the relationships they have with each other. This greatly colors whether the patient will accept a visit from even his or her own children. It may be that some children will be acceptable and others may not. Some religions have separate traditions about boys and girls and how they are treated in family decisions and crisis.

If you don't know how your loved-one will respond to a visit from a child and the patient is not in a position to tell you, talk to the children and ask in an indirect, non-confrontational way if the patient has shielded the children from other big life events. For example, you can ask "has anyone in your family ever been sick in a hospital?" If you know that other family members have been hospitalized, you can ask if the child visited them.

Ultimately, the judgment of whether a patient will benefit from child visitors is up to the family. In most cases it becomes clear either from past experiences or from comments made by the patient to other family members. If you have the entire family weigh in, it is likely you will come up with some consensus.

I will caution you about asking health care workers (doctors and nurses) for opinions about what to do. The only honest answer they can give is that there is no good reason to decide one way or the other from a medical standpoint. If they give you an opinion it is likely going to be their own personal opinion. Since the healthcare workers likely don't know your families as well as you do, take their opinions with a grain of salt.

The worst thing you can do is to force the child to visit if the child is at all reluctant. This is absolutely a lose-lose situation for everyone involved. The child may well be disruptive in trying to express his displeasure or distress, which will certainly affect their own loved one, other patients in the area, and not least, the possibly already harried staff. Such a venture can easily scar the child for life; having a disastrous effect on their own future health care. A child throwing a tantrum at the thought of going to the doctor for even a routine checkup will not be a pleasant experience for anyone.

Will having children in the ICU be disruptive to other patients or healthcare workers?

We have to address this issue only because it has come up in studies of ICU visitation. Particularly, some healthcare workers seem to believe that children in the ICU may be unruly or disruptive. In my experience, this is far from the truth. Children entering my ICU are usually very quiet and orderly. I believe seeing their loved ones in a hospital environment due to the fear of the foreign environment, as well as the anxiety provokes this.

I do encourage only one or two children be allowed to visit at a single time and that an adult accompany each child. If there aren't enough adults to go around, the hospital staff can substitute. I usually have the nurse meet the children and the adults outside of the ICU and explain a little about what they are going to see. In addition, the nurse can outline appropriate behavior in the ICU. Then the adults from the family, the children and nurse can enter the unit together to visit. This seems to ensure that there are no surprises for the children or for the healthcare staff. While in the ICU, I often encourage the children to ask questions and talk to the patient and nurses about what they are feeling. This keeps them focused on what they are doing.

One helpful little hint is to initially turn off the television in the room. Many ICU rooms have televisions that the nurses keep on to have some sound stimulation in the room that is not a beep or buzz. In my experience, children are easily distracted when the television is on. If after the child is visiting for a while and wants to remain in the room, it may be appropriate to turn the TV on to help them pass the time.

Are there realistic risks of children contracting infections in the ICU setting?

I am often asked if it is appropriate to bring children in the ICU due to the infection risk. I have to tell you that I used to be very worried about this. My standard response to families was "The sickest people in the hospital are in the ICUs, therefore, the patients with the worst infections are often in the ICU. Why would you expose your child to this risk?" Interestingly, this idea was based on a number of incorrect assumptions on my part.

First of all, children (except the very young) have immune systems just like adults. In many cases, children haven't yet been exposed to the common bacteria and viruses that can cause disease. However, more and more in ICUs, the viruses and bacteria are selected by the types of antibiotics that we use. Therefore, most adults aren't really exposed to them either. In addition, patients in the ICU are already sick for other reasons, leaving them more than usually susceptible to new or different infections. Healthy people don't usually contract these infections. This is also why healthcare workers seldom contract diseases with which their patients are afflicted.

All of this would suggest that there is little increased risk to children. Prudence would say that any child under the age of 1 year (when their immune systems are still developing) should be kept away from the ICU except for very special circumstances. Any child who has a problem with their immune system either because of a disease they have or because of any medication they take should also be kept from the ICU. (But then, so should any adult visitor under these conditions.) All children should be up to date with their vaccinations. If you choose not to vaccinate your child from childhood diseases, you should probably not have them come and visit.

Finally, there are infectious diseases like tuberculosis and meningitis that are easy to contract. Those patients are usually sequestered in a room with a closed door. Often patients will have to wear masks or other protective equipment to visit. Unfortunately, the masks that are supplied in the hospital don't usually fit children well. If the hospital cannot supply appropriately sized masks and gloves, you should not bring your child into this patient's room.

Hospital visitation policies

There have been almost no studies in the United States about visiting policies for children. Fortunately, many studies have been done in Sweden. Researchers found that when they questioned the nurse managers who are responsible for setting up policies about visitation by children, most had policies regarding visitation by adults but very few had policies concerning children. More disturbing, when asked about whether visitation policies were adhered to, it was clear that most ICUs didn't follow their own policies. Because Europe in general has been more accepting than the United States about family visitation, the findings of this research are quite troubling.

In my experience in four hospital systems, I am not aware of specific policies about children visiting an adult in the ICU. The decision about whether children are allowed is largely left up to the nurse at the patient's bedside. I am not sure if this is a good thing or not. On one level, this personalizes the decision a great deal. The nurse at the bedside has a clear picture of how sick and how interactive a patient is. The nurse may be the most qualified to make the decision about the suitability of child visitation. Yet, I worry about variations in nursing opinions about visitation coloring how children are allowed to visit. It would be unfortunate if a nurse on one day allowed children to visit but another nurse on a subsequent day did not. This can raise fears in children that the patient's condition has worsened. \

If a successful visit has transpired on a given day, you might ask the nurse if this can be made a part of the patient's record. If so, this could ease the way for future visits in case of a change in personnel or other factor in the ICU. Of course, should the patient have an adverse reaction, this might also be noted, for safety's sake.

What do you do if the patient is in serious risk of dying?

If it is a parent who is the patient, and the prognosis is not good, then the other parent or guardian may want to have the child visit to say goodbye. This may be very important for the child to have some closure prior to the death of a parent. Unfortunately, it may also be very traumatic for the child. This is where the benefit to the child must be the first priority. If there is a compelling reason to keep children from visiting, it should be well thought out. I find that the situation where a child's visit is most visibly traumatic is when it is done hastily. Usually, this means a family that has excluded the children from visitation until the prognosis for recovery is found to be grim. The family then hastily brings the children in to visit their parent. The children have had no time to digest what is going on and only a limited knowledge of what has transpired up to that time. Often, the first sign the child has of the severity of the illness is the sight of their loved one in a hospital bed hooked up to tubes and dripping medicines.

In this situation, a child psychologist can be very useful in debriefing the children before and after the visit. It is sometimes possible to have a child psychologist come to the ICU and walk the children through the experience. They can also counsel families about what warning signs to look for to determine if the child has posttraumatic stress disorder or anxiety based on the experience.

I think it is fair to say that our thinking about children visiting the ICU is uninformed. We use our own fears for our children to decide what is best for them. The Pediatric world has studied the interactions of children visiting children and found that they are more observant, more empathetic and more mature than we often give them credit. Although the risks of hurting our children by traumatizing them are real, I think we need to study how children respond to visitation.

One of the points that was brought out by a number of the Swedish investigators was that there are also risks of children not being allowed to visit loved one. When children were asked what was happening to their loved one in the ICU, the responses were more exaggerated and grotesque than was the reality. Sometimes letting children fill in the gaps of what they are not allowed to see with their imagination may be worse than letting them see the reality for themselves.

Chapter 9

The Browns

There were a few hectic days for the Browns, as Olivia slowly began to recover from the big scare. By all accounts, she'd been on the verge of being released from the ICU to a medical wing of the hospital, where she would stay for another few days, building her strength to enable a return to her home. Instead, she was suddenly sicker than she had been, and it took a day or two to discover exactly what had happened to cause the setback.

The culprit was a blood clot that had formed in a vein, due to her inactivity for the time she'd been in the ICU. The clot dislodged itself and traveled to her lung. Fortunately, the monitors to which she was attached signaled the imminent distress, and treatment was immediately put into place. It was a narrow escape. But – even though the long-term prognosis was mostly a good one, the more current situation became vastly different. Certainly, Olivia would be staying in the ICU for another few days, and if all goes well, she would then be sent to the medical wing. After another stay there, she could face rehabilitation in a nursing home-like facility.

"How could this happen?" queried Alex. "Everything was going so well. I don't understand this at all. Did someone make a mistake? How can we find out what happened?" After his initial distress had been alleviated at least somewhat, Alex had a million questions for anyone who would listen to him. His favorite target was Tom, followed closely by Mark. Finally, later the next day, a meeting was arranged with the Intensivist in charge of Olivia's case, as well as Mark, Tom and Alex.

The Intensivist, Dr. Ballard, was not only younger than Alex, but also female, which did not set too well at first, but her calm nature and obvious expertise soon overcame that hurdle. She willingly listened to Alex's questions and proceeded to answer them in a low-key way that Alex could easily understand. "We don't know why these things happen, but since Mrs. Brown was already being monitored, we had a bit of advance warning that something was not quite right. Although the blood clot itself could have been fatal, a more distressing problem was that her oxygen levels dropped to a dangerous level, and this impacted her kidneys. Because that other, younger doctor (Dr. Charles) was in the room at the time of the incident, we were able to circumvent this distress, by immediately increasing Mrs. Brown's oxygen intake, thus eliminating the possible requirement of dialysis, which is uncomfortable and expensive and sometimes on-going."

Alex looked helplessly at Tom, who proceeded to explain what might have been. Mark and the doctor listened carefully; ready to intervene in case of any misinformation. There was none, however, as Tom translated the information perfectly. Alex sat silently for a moment, his eyes closed. He opened them, released a huge sigh and turned to the doctor. "When can she come home?"

"That's hard to say at this time. I don't want to mislead you. I would say that your wife would need to be in hospital here for at least 4 days once she leaves the ICU. She might then need to be in rehab for a while, but it's still too soon to predict that. Regardless of that, however, you must realize that she will not be the energetic wife you knew for perhaps a year. It will take her that long to gain back her strength. If she has no further setbacks, that is. If she becomes ill again, for any reason, it may take even longer. She may even need a wheelchair for a while."

"She will get tired much more quickly, and be unable to perform even the simplest household tasks for a period of several months. She might need assistance in the home, for cooking and cleaning and such."

Alex's heart dropped again. How would he be able to pay for all this? Carolyn was going to grow up much sooner than anyone had anticipated and even Alex, Jr., would be pressed into service, caring more for Ben than he had previously. But – as long as they still had Olivia with them, they would find a way to persevere. They would.

Leaving the ICU

Your time as a family member of an ICU patient is coming to an end. Depending on how the patient fared in the ICU, the transfer out of ICU to a less intense setting may be a good sign ("One step closer to home", as I usually say), or may be a sign that there is no further treatment to allow your family member to reach his or her healthcare goals. Regardless of the outcome, there is one thing that is universal for all family members; just as the patient needs to make a transition from the ICU to a different setting, so does the family.

The first change that many family members notice is that the level of tension decreases as their loved one moves out of the ICU. Initially in the ICU, there is a lot of uncertainty about how well the patient will do. After the initial stages (the first 12 hours) in the ICU, there is still the risk of sudden death throughout the stay. After leaving the ICU, many families tell me that they feel anxious as though there is something missing. When we explore this, we find they are missing the constant tension of the ICU. Over time, that "missing something" feeling goes away as the prognosis becomes more certain and the process of moving out of the hospital to another setting becomes the focus of the family.

Transitions can be very difficult for many people, even if they don't realize it. I recommend professional counseling help for any family member who feels even the slightest hint of sadness or confusion.

There are three possible outcomes to a hospital stay in the ICU: 1) your loved one does well and goes to a hospital ward that is not an ICU, and eventually to home again; 2) your loved one leaves the ICU because there is nothing left that the ICU team can offer to allow him or her to make a suitable recovery; or 3) your loved one passes away. I will take each of these in turn and discuss the special challenges that are associated with each outcome.

Your loved one leaves the ICU

The majority of patients leave the ICU with the prospect of a good recovery. This does not mean that the road ahead will necessarily be an easy one. Many patients still require a prolonged hospital stay after their ICU term is done. In addition, some patients require prolonged admission to rehabilitation facilities. Once home, the road to recovery is long and often involves physical therapy. The transition from the ICU to the regular hospital ward should be a signal that the family's strategy must also change.

The anxiety that most family members feel about their loved one in the ICU causes them to stay close to the hospital. Many of my patient's families stay in the hospital as long as their loved one is in the ICU. Although I don't encourage this as we have talked about earlier, I really worry about families that don't change this tactic when their loved one leaves the ICU. I like to remind families that while the patient is in the ICU, there are nurses, doctors and a lot of other support people taking care of the patient. While I do think that family involvement improves the chances that things won't be overlooked or missed entirely, this constancy comes with a price tag: wearing out the family.

When the patient is no longer in the ICU, there is a real chance that he or she will be coming home in a short time. At home, there are no doctors, nurses or other healthcare workers around all day and night. Family and friends often go back to their normal lives. This leaves one or two family members caring for a person who is still very likely to be dependent for many of his or her activities all day and night. I have had families that have come back to see me months after their loved one came home and said that the hardest transition was when they had to take over the bulk of the management at home. One woman told me that on the day she left the hospital with her husband, she thought she was as tired as she would ever be (even after raising two children). But according to her, that was as nothing compared with how tired she felt a week after her husband had come home.

Understanding the road ahead is most of the battle in this part of the journey. Patients in the ICU have problems associated with the reason they came into the ICU but they may also have problems that originated in the hospital due to their prolonged illness and immobilization (lying in bed). The typical ICU patient, regardless of their illness, leaves the ICU for the hospital ward with three to seven more medicines than they had been taking when they came to the hospital. Some of these medicines will need to be continued when they leave the hospital, some may not be necessary. Eventually, it is likely that your family is going to have to administer these medicines. Understanding what they are and what their side effects are can be very important.

So you can see that your first job as a family member is to become a detective. If your loved one is able to communicate with you effectively, some of this job can go to him or her. I have included a worksheet (worksheet two) to help you in the post-ICU time to organize your thoughts around this. I will discuss each section on the worksheet.

Problem list

The strategy for gathering data can be broken down into two groups I like to call "lumping" and "splitting" (I didn't make up these names, they are used in many circles). Lumping means grouping things together in big categories; for instance, oranges and apples are both fruits with no distinction between them. Splitting, as the name implies is the opposite. Apples can be grouped by color, taste, texture, size and so forth. All of us use a little of both strategies at times depending on the situation. Because of the complexity of illnesses afflicting patients in the ICU, splitting is the better of the two options.

It is important for both you and your loved one to get a clear understanding of what problems you will have to face in the future. I recommend going through a list of symptoms and body regions together so that you don't miss anything. The first list is a list of problems starting from the top down. I list the head, brain, neck, arms, heart, lungs, stomach, personals and legs. In addition, there are common problems that arise in the ICU that have implications for later. Asking the medical team to answer yes or no about these problems can help you anticipate problems down the line. These specific problems that you should ask about are deep vein thrombosis, stomach or intestinal ulcers, pneumonia, delirium, bed sores, diabetes, thyroid problems, asthma, and liver problems. Also ask if your loved one has developed any new allergies to medicines.

I suggest that you give the worksheet to a nurse or doctor and have them fill it out. They can leave blank anything that is not pertinent. When you get it back, you can use the list as a reminder of questions to ask your medical team before leaving the hospital.

Medication list

Having a good medication list that is up to date is very helpful. Medicines are complicated. Many medicines that we use are FDA (Food and Drug Administration) approved, but for indications other than those for which we might commonly use them. For example, aspirin is FDA approved to treat headache and heart disease. We commonly use aspirin for the treatment of stroke and some kinds of blood clots in the legs. If you look at the drug company product information you will not see information about stroke on their literature. Still, the medicine works for stroke.

I suggest that you ask the nurse to list on your paper all the medicines your loved one is taking; a note about whether the patient will need to be on these medicines at home, and what are the indications for each medicine. At this point, the job of the patient and the family is to do some research about the actions and side effects of each medicine so that there are no surprises when you get out of the hospital.

Looking at your home environment

One of the most difficult aspects of getting ready to

leave for home is picturing your loved one (who is still in the hospital) at home. Even if there is a period of time to be spent in rehabilitation, there may still need to be changes made to your home environment. Most hospitals have case managers or social workers that can help you get through some of these questions but, of course, they have no idea of the structure or your home or its contents.

A good exercise is to go to your home and picture yourself with the physical and mental limitations that your loved one has now, not as he used to be. Imagine you are the patient, and go through the important 'little' tasks that we go through every day. How do you get a drink if you are thirsty, go to the bathroom, get to a place for sleeping, get to the telephone, and answer the door? Now, figure out how to make those things possible. Sometimes it may be as simple as rearranging furniture. Other times, it may mean reorganizing your house (moving a second floor bedroom to the first floor). Sometimes it may mean confronting the issue that you need to hire someone (a visiting nurse or aid) to help with some of these functions.

It is true that some of the things you find may change, especially if your loved one will have a prolonged period of rehabilitation. It is sometimes easier to cancel services than to start them in the first place, especially if the need is suddenly urgent. If you find that starting a service or requiring a serious rearrangement in your home may cost money, get as much information as you can about how much it will cost and how long it will take to implement. It will be easier for you to make all this happen if you are not scrambling to find such resources unexpectedly, and at the last minute.

Picking your doctors

In smaller hospitals, you may only see a few doctors who are involved in the care of your loved one. In others, you may see a veritable revolving door of specialists and primary doctors who do a number of weeks on a hospital service tending to the patients there and then pass the service on to a colleague in their group. This gives you the opportunity to choose the physicians you will deal with later. I find it humorous at times that there is such a lot written about carefully choosing your doctors in the outpatient clinic, but little attention is paid to the fact that most patients in the hospital are assigned the doctor who first saw them, possibly even in the Emergency Department (the first come, first serve system). If you find a doctor with whom you have a good relationship, ask if he or she would be willing to see you as an outpatient. The same thing goes with specialists. Pick the ones who gave you the most trusted advice and those with whom you had the best relationship.

Rehabilitation

Many patients need a period of focused physical and cognitive (memory) therapy before going home. Rehabilitation offers this in a live-in setting that allows patients to get more hours of structured activity than would be available as a home patient coming to the outpatient physical therapy clinic. In some diseases like a stroke of the brain and heart attack, aggressive rehabilitation has been one of the most important advances in therapy over the last 50 years. Knowing how to pick a rehabilitation facility is difficult. It depends on the physical ability of your loved one, your insurance policy, the availability of beds at the various rehabilitation facilities when your loved one is ready, the expertise of the facility and the distance from your home.

There are two levels of rehabilitation based on the tolerance for exercise. To qualify for "Acute Rehabilitation", the patient has to be able to do a total of three hours of therapy per day. This may seem like a manageable amount of therapy but this can be a daunting task for someone who has been seriously ill, and in a bed for more than a week.

The biggest advantage of acute rehabilitation is that rehabilitation facilities are regulated by a federal agency that evaluates them every couple of years to make sure they meet certain minimum requirements. This means that regardless of the facility, there is a level of security in knowing that they are accredited. In addition, some facilities have special expertise in one type of rehabilitation. For example, there are a few centers that specialize in the treatment of patients with spinal cord injuries.

Certain insurance policies make contracts with specific rehabilitation centers and ask that their clients go to these facilities. In addition, the demand for rehabilitation has increased steadily over the last 20 years. We are still in a situation where every patient has the ability to go to the appropriate level of rehabilitation but the choice of location may depend on the availability of beds at any particular facility. If there is availability in multiple places, it only makes sense to find one close to your home so that you can visit more frequently.

If your loved one doesn't qualify for acute rehabilitation, there are a number of facilities that we refer to as "subacute rehabilitation". This offers some of the advantages to a nursing home setting but doesn't require the three hours of daily therapy. The best way to think about subacute rehabilitation is a nursing home that can provide some physical therapy.

Nursing Home

At the other end of the spectrum of rehabilitation is what most people call a nursing home. Long term care facilities (the socially appropriate name) are places where people who are unable to care for themselves at home go to get the care they need on a chronic basis. Many people have strong fears about being left all alone in a nursing home when they get sick or old. Although this may occur, this sort of facility is also appropriate for someone who has been in the ICU and needs more time to recover and build up strength in order to qualify for acute rehabilitation. This person may well end up in a nursing home for a short stay.

All of the insurance and location issues that are important for rehabilitation will also pertain to nursing homes. I will warn you that not all nursing homes are alike. Almost more than every other level of care in medicine, there are significant differences between facilities. The only good way to evaluate them is to visit each possibility. I recommend that someone from the family physically go to the nursing home and meet with the staff and the patients. A good rule of thumb is that if you don't find your visit tolerable, living there will be even worse.

There are a number of models of care that have been developed to give patients as much autonomy as possible. Assisted living arrangements where residents still have a residence to call their own but are supervised by nurses has changed the landscape of long-term care for some patients who are too sick to go home but are able to care for themselves in a limited way. Unfortunately, these alternative nursing options can be expensive and are not generally covered as well by insurance companies as other types of nursing home facilities.

Permanent changes

Many family members come to me in the course of an ICU stay and ask, "When will our lives get back to normal?" For some, the answer may be 'never'. Some diseases that bring people to the ICU leave obvious permanent damage; an example of this is stroke. But even diseases like pneumonia that leave no signs of permanent damage by x-ray or laboratory tests often take a toll on both the patient and the family. For some families it is as simple as the realization that life is fragile. In other cases, long ICU stays can lead to deconditioning of the muscles and damage to the psyche (depression or anxiety). It is important to NOT have all your hopes and dreams based on the assumption that everything will eventually be all right.

A friend of mine who is a psychologist once told me about a circle model of human goals. Let me explain this. He said that at any point in our lives, we look at ourselves, and what we are capable of, and use that information to make decisions about what goals to pursue. For example, if a person is very good at fixing cars and really likes mechanical things, he or she may choose a goal of owning a car repair shop. It is unlikely that the same person would set a goal of becoming a doctor. Throughout our lives, as our aptitudes become clearer, we set goals based on what we know about ourselves. Interestingly, much of what we think of as aptitudes are not our physical abilities but our life circumstances. How many times can you remember your grandmother or grandfather saying not everyone had the money to go to college. This was a circumstance of that era. However, as we grow older and act on our goals, it becomes harder and harder to change our perception of ourselves.

When we have an illness that alters our abilities, the obvious thing to do is to alter our goals. But what if the illness limits our abilities to do our chosen profession? I (JP) for one would be heartbroken if an illness caused me to lose the ability to be a doctor. The same goes for many people. For this reason, many patients continue to strive to keep the same goals they had when they were healthier.

Yet, as hard as it sounds, changing our goals is *exactly* what we need to do. And it is not just the patient, but also the whole family that needs to reevaluate their situation. If you are the spouse of a patient who was in the ICU with an illness that caused permanent disability, you may not have the ability to go back to work full-time or take that promotion because your life circumstances will no longer allow it.

Unfortunately, I have not been able to find any good resources – other than professional counseling – to help with this journey. It must be very difficult to have to reevaluate your situation and make new goals especially if those new realistic goals are considered a step down in prestige, money or independence. Social workers in hospitals can help, as can clergy. Sometimes, consulting with a financial counselor can fill in some of the questions about how much money your family needs to live and cover medical expenses. I wish someone would develop a resource for families to address realistic goal setting.

The challenges of being the caregiver

It is assumed that being the spouse or life partner of a sick patient means that you will, of necessity, be the primary caregiver when the patient goes home from the hospital. Unsurprisingly, being a caregiver for a sick patient is a big undertaking. Many people take the stance that life is unpredictable but you just have to make do (if life gives you lemons, make lemonade). Others find this transition harder to rationalize. I recommend that all primary caregivers seek out professional help in the form of a counselor, clergy member or close friend to support them during this time. Feeling isolated is the first sign of impending problems.

Losing the sick role

The last issue that needs to be raised about the transition out of the ICU to the regular hospital ward is the issue of the relationship you have with your loved one. When someone experiences a life-threatening event, it is common for spouse, children and friends to treat the sick person as one would treat a child. This is very appropriate when the patient is incapacitated. It is always amusing to me to notice how quickly and easily we slip into the role of protector and provider and how hard it is to then get back to the original role of child or spouse.

It isn't just families that have a hard time changing – or adjusting – their roles. After getting used to having a nurse or assistant do everything for them, sometimes the patient has a hard time reverting to some independence. When you add this to self-doubts and fears about the future, it is not hard to see why some patients may have trouble getting out of the 'invalid' role.

As hard as it may seem, it is truly a more healthy psychological option to help your loved one move out of the sick role as quickly as is feasible. The risk comes from pushing too hard and possibly overwhelming your loved one. It is a fine balance between coddling too long and pushing too hard. Most families who are conscious of this dilemma get the mix right. Families who don't recognize this as a challenge often do not.

The ICU doctors find there is nothing more they can offer your loved one

There are times when, no matter how good our current level of science is, we simply cannot help a patient. This can happen when the disease process that is affecting your loved one cannot be adequately treated by current therapies. In other cases, the treatments, although possibly effective, will leave the patient so debilitated that it doesn't make sense to start. Finally, some patients have strong beliefs about having heroic measures taken that may prolong life but won't necessarily improve the quality of life.

Regardless of the reason, there are times in the care of patients when the ICU is simply not the right setting to continue their care. This doesn't mean that care ends for the patient. I often tell families that when we decide that ICU care is not the right treatment path, all we are saying is that our care strategy has shifted from our current path to another. In the ICU, the overriding goal is to save lives at all cost. When saving life at any cost isn't in the best interest of the patient, we change the goal of therapy. Usually this means focusing our goal on comfort measures instead of life-saving measures.

Comfort care

No physician, nurse, or other healthcare provider is naïve enough to think we can cure all disease. I personally believe that we can TREAT all patients. For those that can be helped, we help; for those that cannot be, we can offer comfort. Many people associate comfort care with hastening death in patients (called euthanasia). This misconception is understandable. As part of the comfort care of most patients, we prescribe medicines (particularly morphine) that if given in overdose can lead to death. In other countries where "assisted suicide" is legal, this is often the case. In the United States, the government and the medical community have decided that any attempt to hasten death is unacceptable medical care.

Many families also have the misconception that comfort care is always the same regimen. I overheard one wife tell a brother-in-law that her husband "got switched to the comfort care, so he will be getting that." I find that not everyone's comfort level is the same. When patients can answer for themselves, the question of what make them comfortable can be easily answered. If patients are unable to speak or are incapable of understanding the issue, we rely on families to guide us based on what they know about their loved one.

The third misconception about comfort care is that it always means less care. It is true that when our goals change, many of the medicines are discontinued. However, I have performed some of the most extravagant and invasive procedures to make patients comfortable.

A good example of this occurred when I was in my residency training. There was a man of about 50 years of age who had a progressive and ultimately lethal breathing condition. When we decided that there was nothing more we could do to improve his lungs and get him home, we (the patient, his family and the medical team) made the decision to change our goal to comfort. I asked him what he felt would make him comfortable. He told me that he wanted to see his granddaughter before he died. She was four, and lived across the country. I told him the only way to get to that goal was to put a breathing tube into his windpipe and breath for him until she could get here. He said that he absolutely didn't want to die on a breathing machine. We tried some machines that move air in and out to the lung from the outside of the body, but they didn't do enough.

I thought we were at an impasse until one day, during lunch with one of my mentors – an older neurologist who was getting ready to retire – I told him about my dilemma. He said, "That's easy, put him in an iron lung (an old time breathing machine from the 1920's that they used for patients with polio)". I told him I was sure we didn't have an iron lung. At the next table over, one of the doctors said, "Sure, we have an iron lung. We use it for a historical display from time to time". I made a few phone calls to make sure it still worked, and put my patient in the iron lung for three days. His granddaughter was able to visit and spend a whole day with him. The next day, with his entire family present, he said good-bye, we turned off the machine and he died peacefully. The most memorable part of this experience for me was that before we stopped the iron lung, he thanked me. I will never forget the day that a patient whom I couldn't save thanked me. It has since happened a few more times, and although I hate it when patients die, I take special pride in knowing that I can – and will – treat even the most terminally ill patients.

Palliative care

Some patients who are in the ICU have problems or diseases for which more ICU treatment is not going to be helpful. This is not to say that they are going to die immediately. In this situation, it is often useful to have a group of healthcare workers (doctors, nurses, social workers, etc.) who can help patients who have longer-term terminal diseases. Over the last 15-20 years, this group has gelled into a specialty called "palliative care". Their role is to treat symptoms associated with terminal and chronic diseases when the goal of therapy is to comfort.

Because of the relative newness of this group, we as intensive care doctors are still figuring out ways to interact with palliative care services in many hospitals. It then becomes the job of the family to remind the ICU doctors to call palliative care when leaving the ICU. As a group, they have been very successful at making patients more comfortable. They also do a great deal of research on this subject which means that new advances in comfort management will come from these practitioners.

Hospice

A separate but intertwined service is Hospice. This is the traditional service that was initially developed for cancer patients so that they could spend their last days at home. Many hospice services remain as only homebound therapy but some more progressive hospice services now offer services for hospitalized patients. Their purpose is to make the end of life more comfortable. Sometimes this means prescribing and dispensing medicines; sometimes it is as simple as coming into the house and washing the clothes.

Preparing yourself

Lastly, if treatments for your loved one are not going to improve their outcome and they are destined to die, then it is important to prepare yourself. Many people feel that such preparation means getting all the finances and paperwork in order. I think it is much more important to prepare yourself emotionally for the loss of your loved one. Life without a loved one can very lonely. Often after a prolonged illness, especially if your loved one has been suffering, death can be a relief. Many times, family members whose loved one had passed away in the hospital come back and tell me that they still feel guilty for having felt relief that their loved one had died.

I feel compelled to tell you a word about time. It is exceedingly difficult to gauge how quickly a patient will die once aggressive therapy is discontinued. My personal belief (although this is not something that medical science can endorse) is that the patient's own will to live is supremely important. Families tell me over and over that their family member seemed to lose their will to live prior to dying. If you ask the doctor "how long will my loved one live?" after a change of strategy to comfort care, the best answer is still only a guess. For example, the last time I tried to answer this question, I stated that the patient would probably not last more than a few minutes. After we discontinued the ventilator support, the patient remained in a coma but survived for seven more days. Needless to say, I don't usually offer time predictions anymore.

PROBLEM LIST	MEDICATION LIST AND PHYSICIANS	HOME, REHAB AND NURSING HOME
		Things to change at home
1	1	1
2	2	2
3	3	3
4	4	4
5	5	5
6	6	Possible Rehabilitation Facilities and Nursing Homes
7	7	1
8	8	2
	9	3
	10	4
	Follow-up care	Support Services for Caregivers:
	Physician — Office Phone Number	
	1	
	2	
	3	
	4	

Chapter 10

What if -- ? Sharing the Grief

Father Malone had trained and been ordained as a parish priest. He was an intellectually curious man, always interested in learning new things, and happily accepted an offer by a local hospital to be a hospital chaplain. Within a year, he discovered this to be his 'true calling'. He was astonished by the amount of information that was thrown at both patients and their families, most of which, being in 'hospital-speak' was not readily understood by non-medical persons.

He set out to educate himself in these matters, and found himself the 'go-to' chaplain, serving people of all ages and races – and faiths. Every encounter left him more certain than ever that he was in the right place at the right time, and he began to educate himself in those areas in which he felt he could make the most difference.

Now, several years later, he had acquired some legal knowledge, some medical knowledge, but mostly he increased his people skills, by knowing where to find the information needed by families at the most crucial period of their lives. He had made a sort of specialty regarding the especially thorny topics of 'end of life' matters.

Thus, when Olivia's very life seemed to be most at risk, he was able to consult and console her family. His warmth and concern provided a bridge for them, and he had barely scratched the surface of the 'what if --?' topics, when the happy news arrived that her condition had stabilized. He was overjoyed to find his extensive knowledge was now not needed. Happily, he returned all the sample papers he had brought with him back to the folders from whence they came.

When your loved one dies

Despite all of our best intentions, some patients still die. When this happens, there are a few unassailable facts that families have to face, and I have put them in a short list:
1) You and your family are going to survive.
2) There needs to be a period of mourning.
3) There are some administrative tasks that need to be completed.
4) A benefit (and comfort) for many families is finding a way to memorialize their loved one.

As defeated as you will feel when you hear that your loved one has died, there are some real steps you can take to help ease the transition from mourning to continuing life even though it is drastically changed by your loved one's absence.

Often after a prolonged illness, especially if your loved one has been suffering, death can be a relief. Many times, family members whose loved one had passed away in the hospital come back and tell me that they still feel guilty for having felt relief when their loved one died.

It is very common after the death of a relative following a complicated illness in the ICU to experience a number of emotions competing against each other. It is not uncommon for families to feel sadness, happiness, relief, loneliness, desperation, anger, and hatred all at the same time. When a patient dies, taking a few minutes to exploring these emotions with other members of your family can often lead to a better transition to life afterwards.

Decisions to make

When a patient dies in the hospital, the family grieves and collects to support each other. At no other time in the daily life of a hospital does a family so totally block out what is going on around them as when a patient first dies. I have spoken to family members weeks after a loved one died and they often tell me that they don't remember anything from the time they were given the news until after they'd left the hospital.

Unfortunately, there are some issues that need to be resolved prior to the family leaving the hospital. I recommend that the family designate a member with enough knowledge of the patient and the family's wishes to answer the questions and fill out the paperwork. In my experience, this is often a son-in-law or close family friend. This takes some of the burden of having to answer questions away from the wife, children, or closest loved one.

Usually, there are administrators whose job it is to collect all the data necessary for the death certificate, hospital forms and requests for special services (which will be discussed below). In our hospital, we have a family liaison service that supports families of patients who are severely ill. When a patient dies, the family liaison (who likely already knows the family) meets with the family in a quiet room to discuss these issues. Although many hospitals do not have the resources to support an individual program to support family in such times, they may have other suggestions to offer. It's always good to inquire.

Autopsy

Autopsy has become synonymous with the removal of organs after a patient dies. Most of us over the age of 40 associate this with the scene in the opening credits of the television show, *Quincy* from the 1970's. Although the examination of the body is an important part of an autopsy, the term actually means an investigation into the cause of a patient's death. This includes a close review of the patient's history before entering the hospital, an evaluation of laboratory data and clinical records from the hospital stay, and an examination of the body including microscopic examination of tissues.

We offer autopsies to families as a service. Many families want to know the actual cause of death. This is especially true if the cause of death could possibly be due to a genetic condition that can be inherited by children of the patient. Physicians also appreciate autopsies because we get a chance to really investigate the cause of death of the patient in a way that our tests in living patients cannot investigate. In our hospital, all families are asked whether they would like an autopsy done.

Coroner

The coroner's office in every county reserves the right to investigate the death of any patient who dies in suspicious circumstances. This can be distressing for families who believe that their loved one has died due to an illness that was nobody's fault. It can be shocking when a loved one dies of, for instance, cardiac arrest after a long illness and the family is told that the hospital cannot release the body to the family but must instead send the body to the coroner's office for further evaluation. This can be particularly stressful for people who have religious beliefs that involve strict burial rites.

"Suspicious circumstances" can be a confusing concept for families who are interested in just getting their family member's body to a funeral home and making preparations for the funeral. In our county, we have strict guidelines about what constitutes a suspicious circumstance. The goal of these guidelines is to make sure that the coroner's office doesn't miss any potential criminal activity. Therefore, any patient in a coma who is brought to the hospital from home or a nursing home and doesn't regain consciousness prior to their demise (regardless of the cause of the coma) is an automatic referral to the coroner's office. Likewise, any patient who goes to surgery awake and doesn't regain consciousness prior to death is automatically referred to the coroner.

An illustrative example of how this can cause an innocent situation to require a coroner's inquest is a family that I met as their loved one was admitted to the ICU after a cardiac arrest at home. This man was known to have a very bad heart with a number of heart attacks. His cardiologist had recommended that he have an implantable defibrillator placed to treat possible arrhythmias. The patient, with the understanding of his family, chose not to put in the defibrillator. When he had an arrhythmia that left him with a rapidly terminal illness, the family was actually expecting this outcome. They were very surprised when I told them that the body had to go the coroner's office for an inquiry due to the fact that he was unconscious at home and never regained consciousness. The family felt strongly that they didn't want an autopsy. We had to inform the family that the coroner was entitled to do whatever evaluation he might find appropriate. Luckily, after discussion with the coroner, he agreed not to do a surgical autopsy for this patient.

(Note: each county has its own method for determining actions by the Coroner. Some Coroners are elected, some appointed; some are doctors, some are not. The rules governing one county may differ greatly from the adjacent county. If you have questions regarding your own county, or the county in which your loved one is hospitalized, ask the local doctor in charge.)

In today's scattered world, when almost nobody stays in one place for a lifetime, it's likely that many of your family members live in other states or even countries. The pressure of caring for a loved one during a terminal illness is much greater than many people immediately recognize. When it then becomes necessary to plan a funeral, the pressures increase exponentially, leaving everyone unhappy, unsatisfied, and feeling very fragmented. This is especially true for far-flung family members who may not be able to get home in a timely fashion.

A growing trend is to have a very small, private service for only those family members and close friends who are in the immediate area. Then, a month or two later, when travel between home and away can be coordinated with less strain for all concerned, a memorial service can be held. In this situation, it is easier to remember the loved one in happier times, and in many cases provides for a reunion of sorts, based around these more joyful memories.

Some religions require an immediate burial, and a celebration of the loved one's life at a later date can be a helpful first step towards healing for all concerned.

Giving something back

Many families have difficulty finding good in the death of a loved one. I have noticed that the families who have made the best peace with the death of a loved one (especially a young person) found some way to give something back to the community or a cause about which the loved one felt strongly. A bench at the botanical garden or a donation to a children's charity can be very healing. In my hometown, my physics teacher lost his wife suddenly to a brain aneurysm. He established a charity in her name and had a charity golf tournament to raise funds. He told me that not only did this help him to heal, but was also very helpful in assisting his young children to cope with the loss of their mother.

Epilogue

The Browns a year later

Olivia was unaccustomed to being ill, but the time she spent in the ICU made a believer out of her. Once she was able to leave the ICU, she spent another week in the regular medical ward. From there she went to rehab for a week, before finally being released to return to her home. She looked and felt more like her grandmother than herself, and was grumpy and grouchy, even when her family was there. This, in turn, made her feel even worse. She was occasionally weepy, until finally she confessed to Alex, "I was so frightened! I didn't want to leave you . . . and the kids."

Having no experience at being ill, neither she nor her family realized that it would take a while for her to feel good again. Even after two months, when she began to look more like her old self again, she still did not have the strength she'd had before the illness. This added to her depression.

At four months, it was hard to tell just by looking at her that she'd ever been ill, but those who knew her could easily see that she still moved more slowly and carefully than before. She began to worry that she would never regain her strength. To her surprise, the visit to her doctor was very reassuring. Especially when he told her that it would take a while for her to feel good again. He added, "Don't worry about it, take your time. There's no target date for you to feel great again. I think it's pretty safe to say you should not have any long-term effects. BUT –" and here, he shook his finger at her in a gentle reprimand, "don't ever do this to yourself again. You are a precious, integral part of your family. They need you, they love you and they want you to stay with them for many years to come. You must take care of yourself first, and only then, will you be able to take care of your family."

It was a boost to her confidence to be told she didn't

have to return again until one year had passed. Olivia learned to take care of herself, and even to rest now and then. She began to teach her daughter some of the things a good wife and mother should know. And, occasionally, her son sat in on the lessons. Slowly, life became more livable.

The doctor was pleasantly surprised to see this vibrant, healthy and cheerful woman stride into his office. Her confidence had not just returned, but increased, as well.

Olivia smiled as she told him of her current activities, now that she'd regained her strength. "Thank you for saving my life," she told him. "It's so much more precious to me now. My children and my husband join with me in saying a heartfelt 'Thank you!'"

In Closing

The road through the ICU is terrifying for patients but sometimes I think it is more terrifying for families. How many times do you hear sports stars say they are more nervous watching a game than playing in it? I think it is the lack of control that ultimately makes it so difficult.

Over the last 40 years, patients in the ICU have survived more of their illnesses every year. Some of this is attributable to better surgical technique and better post-hospitalization rehabilitation but I would like to think that some of this improvement is also based on good intensive care. I wonder at the advances we have made and how well patients who really should have died have survived.

The new focus of research in the ICU is not just saving lives but making sure that life has quality. There are a number of occasions where patients have come back to see me alive and apparently well after an ICU stay where I thought for sure they were going to die. After feeling very good about myself, I realize that their life challenges are great and they struggle. Measuring the things we do that save lives is easy but it is just as important to measure which of those interventions or medications also improve the lives of the patients who survive.

As a final anecdote, I will tell you about a patient who did both; he survived and survived well. He was a 17-year-old young man I saw in the ICU as part of my training who was getting ready for his high school prom when one of his friends offered him some drugs. He had never tried drugs before but on his prom, he thought "What the heck". He began having seizures that night that got progressively worse until the only way we could control them was to put him in a medication induced coma. Even then, he would have seizures a few times a day. Unable to control his seizures for 3 weeks, our team sat down with his mom and told her that he likely wouldn't live but that we could try one more thing, a deep coma. The chances he would come out mentally normal were slim and he would likely face a lot of complications from his ICU stay. After a more aggressive and risky treatment, the seizures stopped and he experienced every complication an ICU patient can have from infections to blood clots to bedsores. We diligently treated each problem as it occurred.

I am not sure if the treatment helped or his seizures just ran their course but he remained in the ICU for three more weeks until he was well enough to go to rehabilitation. He has lived long enough for me to get very nice announcements about his college graduation and his wedding. If we could bottle whatever we did for that young man and use it for all of our patients, our goal would be achieved.

There is tragedy that occurs in the ICU to be sure, but I am always amazed at how many sport teams, amusement parks and Vegas shows use the expression "this is where miracles happen". They should spend a month with me to see where miracles happen. My goals in the ICU are very simple; fix who we can fix, comfort when we can't cure, and treat everyone as best we can and with the dignity they deserve. I am pretty confident that almost the complete majority of doctors, nurses, nutritionists, pharmacists, physical, speech and occupational therapist, and environmental specialists in intensive care units around the world feel the same way I do.

If this book was purchased because you have a loved one in the ICU, I truly hope it was a help and a comfort to you. I also hope your loved one made it through this ordeal healthy and will be soon returning home to you. If your loved one was not so fortunate, I hope they were treated with care and compassion. Of all my jobs (JP): physician, researcher, administrator, teacher, husband and father, I am very surprised that the title I think may make the biggest impact to people (through this book) is author. I am very thankful for this opportunity.

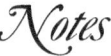

Notes

Notes